Small Animal
Orthopaedics
The Hindlimb

Copyright © 2020 Grupo Asís Biomedia, SL
Plaza Antonio Beltrán Martínez n° 1, planta 8 - letra I
(Centro empresarial El Trovador)
50002 Zaragoza - Spain

First printing: January 2020

Illustrator:
Jacob Gragera Artal

ISBN: 978-84-17640-71-2
DL: Z 2178-2019

Design, layout and printing:
Grupo Asís Biomedia, SL
www.grupoasis.com
info@grupoasis.com

Warning:

Veterinary science is constantly evolving, as are pharmacology and the other sciences. Inevitably, it is therefore the responsibility of the veterinary surgeon to determine and verify the dosage, the method of administration, the duration of treatment and any possible contraindications to the treatments given to each individual patient, based on his or her professional experience. Neither the publisher nor the author can be held liable for any damage or harm caused to people, animals or properties resulting from the correct or incorrect application of the information contained in this book.

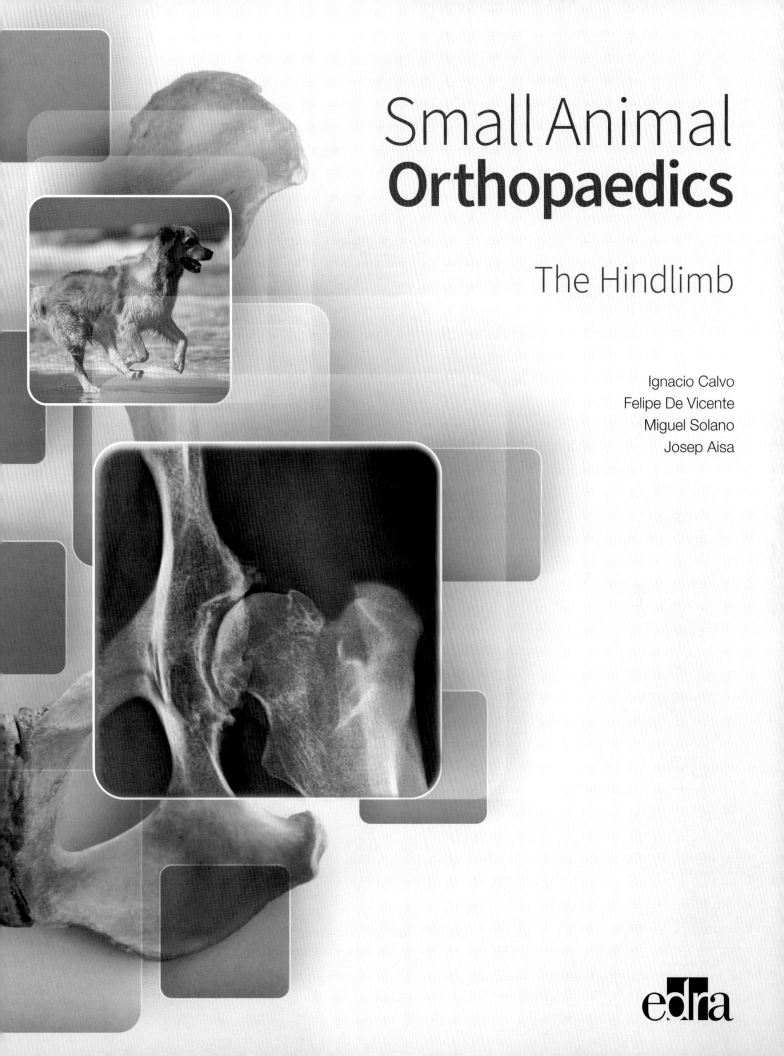

Small Animal
Orthopaedics

The Hindlimb

Ignacio Calvo
Felipe De Vicente
Miguel Solano
Josep Aisa

edra

THE AUTHORS

IGNACIO CALVO

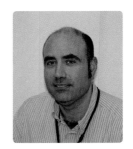

Ignacio graduated in veterinay medicine from the University of Córdoba (Spain) in 2000. After a training period at the Complutense University of Madrid, he undertook a rotating internship and residency in small animal surgery (orthopaedics) at the University of Glasgow (United Kingdom). He was awarded the RCVS (Royal College of Veterinary Surgeons) Certificate in Small Animal Surgery (CertSAS) in 2009 and the European Diploma in Small Animal Surgery (Dipl. ECVS) in 2012. In 2016 he received his PhD from the Complutense University of Madrid for his work on the tibial tuberosity advancement procedure. Ignacio has worked at Glasgow and Dublin veterinary schools, the Royal Veterinary College and at Fitzpatrick Referrals (UK). He is currently the Head of Orthopaedic Surgery at Hospital Veterinario Vetsia in Leganés, Madrid. He is the musculoskeletal section editor of *BMC Veterinary Research* (impact factor 1.9), as well as a member of the AOVET European board and the AOVET international education commission.

FELIPE DE VICENTE

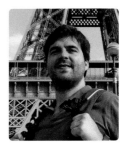

Felipe graduated in veterinary medicine from the Complutense University of Madrid (Spain) in 2003 and was awarded a PhD from the same university in 2009. He completed a rotating internship at Glasgow University in 2008 and a small animal surgery residency at University College Dublin in 2012. He was awarded the European Diploma in Small Animal Surgery from the European College of Veterinary Surgeons (ECVS) in 2014, and became an RCVS-recognised specialist in this discipline in 2016. Felipe has been Lecturer in Small Animal Surgery at the University of Glasgow, he has worked as a surgery specialist at Caldervets hospital (Yorkshire, England), and has also been Senior Lecturer and Head of Service of the Orthopaedics Department at the University of Liverpool. Since September 2018 he has been working as a specialist in surgery at Pride Veterinary Centre (Derby, England) and Hospital Veterinario Puchol (Madrid, Spain).

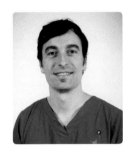

MIGUEL SOLANO

Miguel graduated in veterinary medicine from the Autonomous University of Barcelona (Spain) in 2007. After a year working in a referral emergency centre in Barcelona, he moved to the UK in July 2008 where he undertook a surgical internship at Fitzpatrick Referrals, gaining extensive experience in all aspects of small animal orthopaedics and neurosurgery. Following his interest in small animal surgery, he moved to Cambridge to take up a one-year junior training scholarship at the University of Cambridge before completing a three-year European College of Veterinary Surgeons–approved residency programme in small animal surgery at Fitzpatrick referrals and VRCC (UK). Miguel became a diplomate of the ECVS in February 2015. He continues to work as a senior clinician at Fitzpatrick Referrals combining a very busy case load with clinical research.

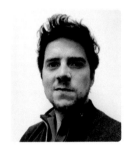

JOSEP AISA

Josep graduated in veterinary medicine from the Autonomous University of Barcelona in 1999. After several years working as a small animal veterinary surgeon in Spain and the UK, in 2007 he undertook a rotating internship at Davies Veterinary Specialists in the UK. He completed his residency in small animal surgery at University College Dublin (Ireland) in 2014. Josep joined the University of Glasgow's School of Veterinary Medicine (Scotland, 2014–2017) as both a lecturer and clinical specialist in the Small Animal Surgery Service. He then spent some time as a specialist in private practice before joining the University of Tennessee in 2019. He is recognised by the RCVS and the European Board of Veterinary Specialisation (EBVS) as a European Veterinary Specialist in Small Animal Surgery (Dipl. ECVS).

PREFACE

Small Animal Orthopaedics. The Hindlimb has been conceived as a practical book in which the text and images are equally important. It focuses on the most common diseases affecting the hindlimbs of cats and dogs and how they can be treated surgically.

This book has been divided into three main chapters, in which the different diseases and their surgical treatments are described according to the joint they affect: the hip, the stifle and the tarsus.

The purpose of this work, and therefore the aspect on which we the authors have placed special emphasis, is to provide a clear description of the different surgical techniques, since none of the books published to date in this field shows them in detail. Each description includes the following sections: introduction, indications, surgical planning, surgical technique, postoperative management, outcome and complications. In those cases in which several techniques may be used for the surgical treatment of a disease, such as hip dysplasia or cranial cruciate ligament disease, a section on the key aspects of the disease is also included. All the descriptions are accompanied by pictures of the procedures for readers to better understand how these are performed.

We believe this book will be useful to both less experienced surgeons taking their first steps in the field and veterinary surgeons with previous experience in orthopaedics.

The authors

TABLE OF CONTENTS

01
THE HIP

INTRODUCTION

The hip (coxofemoral) joint has a wide range of motion due to its ball and socket configuration; it allows flexion, extension, abduction, adduction, as well as internal and external rotation. Congruity between the acetabulum and the femoral head is necessary to enable a smooth, pain-free range of motion and normal transmission of forces through the hip joint. Surgical conditions of the hip include hip dysplasia, Legg–Calvé–Perthes disease, hip luxation, acetabular fractures, and femoral head or neck fractures.

The surgical approach to the hip must be large enough to visualise the articular cartilage and the shape of the femoral head and acetabulum, as decision-making during the surgery might be influenced by the changes found during the procedure.

STANDARD APPROACH TO THE HIP JOINT

Several surgical approaches to the hip have been described (Johnson, 2014). Most surgical procedures are performed through a standard craniolateral approach. A skin incision is made in a linear or curvilinear fashion, starting 2–3 cm craniodorsal to the greater trochanter of the femur and extending distally along the cranial border of the proximal third of the femur (Fig. 1).

The subcutaneous tissue is dissected until the biceps femoris muscle is identified, with its muscle fibres running in a proximocaudal to distocranial direction (Fig. 2). The fascia lata attaches along the cranial aspect of the biceps femoris muscle. An incision is made in the superficial leaf of the fascia lata, immediately cranial to the biceps femoris muscle, and extended proximally and distally. Access to the deep leaf of the fascia lata is achieved by retracting the biceps femoris muscle caudally (Fig. 3).

The deep leaf of the fascia lata can be followed proximally to find the tensor fasciae latae muscle and the superficial gluteal muscle (Fig. 4).

The deep leaf of the fascia lata is incised from distal to proximal, continuing between the tensor fasciae latae and superficial gluteal muscles (Fig. 5). Gelpi retractors are very useful to maintain the dissection planes by retracting the fascia lata and tensor fasciae latae muscle cranially and the biceps femoris muscle caudally. These Gelpi retractors need to be placed gently to avoid any injury to the sciatic nerve.

The vastus lateralis muscle, which originates on the craniolateral aspect of the femoral neck, is located immediately underneath the fascia lata (Fig. 6). In certain procedures, it is necessary to perform a partial elevation of the medial aspect of the origin of the vastus lateralis muscle at the femoral neck. The middle gluteal muscle is identified underneath the superficial gluteal muscle, inserting on the greater trochanter of the femur. The middle gluteal muscle is retracted proximally with a hand-held retractor such as a Langenbeck retractor (Fig. 7) to expose the deep gluteal muscle.

The deep gluteal muscle is easily identified inserting on the cranial aspect of the greater trochanter, with its fibres running in a cranioproximal direction. A partial tenotomy of the tendon of the deep gluteal muscle can be performed to visualise the hip joint capsule underneath (Fig. 8). The deep gluteal tenotomy usually involves transecting one third to half of the width of the tendon and continuing cranioproximally through the deep gluteal muscle, following the direction of the muscle fibres (L-shape incision). This tenotomy must be performed approximately 2 mm away from the tendon insertion to allow resuturing of the tendon during surgical closure. In chronic hip conditions, it is common to find adhesions between the joint capsule and the deep gluteal muscle; these can be severed by a combination of sharp and blunt dissection if needed.

In those conditions in which it is still intact (such as hip dysplasia and Legg–Calvé–Perthes disease), the joint capsule is then incised in an inverted T-shape to facilitate closure after the surgical procedure (Fig. 9). The incision can be continued if needed, with partial elevation of the medial aspect of the vastus lateralis muscle insertion using a sharp blade or periosteal elevator to help visualise the neck of the femur.

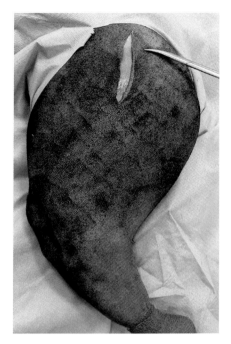

Figure 1. Skin incision along the cranial border of the femur, starting 2–3 cm craniodorsal to the greater trochanter and extending distally along the proximal third of the femur. The surgeon is using Metzenbaum scissors to indicate the position of the greater trochanter of the femur, the landmark for the skin incision.

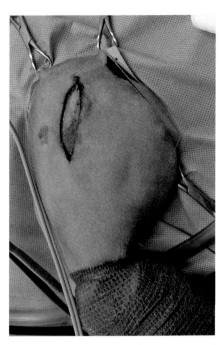

Figure 2. Exposure of the biceps femoris muscle and subcutaneous tissue.

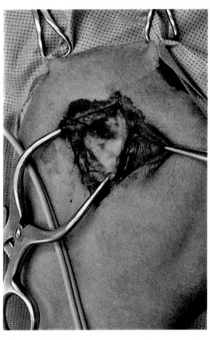

Figure 3. Gelpi retractors are used to retract the subcutaneous tissue. The biceps femoris muscle is located caudally (star), while the fascia lata is located cranial to the biceps femoris muscle. In the image, the tensor fasciae latae muscle can be seen at the most craniodorsal aspect of the fascia lata (arrow).

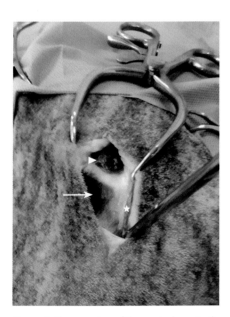

Figure 4. Close-up view of the surgical approach. The deep leaf of the fascia lata is attached to the cranial aspect of the biceps femoris muscle (star). The tensor fasciae latae muscle (arrow) and the superficial gluteal muscle (arrowhead) are located proximal to the deep leaf of the fascia lata as shown in this image.

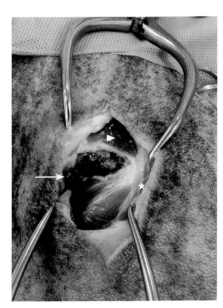

Figure 5. An incision has been made in the fascia lata, just cranial to the biceps femoris muscle (star), and extended proximally between the tensor fasciae latae muscle (arrow) and the superficial gluteal muscle (arrowhead).

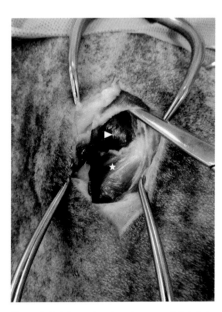

Figure 6. Gelpi retractors have been used distally to retract the biceps femoris muscle caudally and the tensor of the fasciae latae muscle cranially. The vastus lateralis muscle (star) can be seen underneath this surgical plane. The surgeon is retracting the superficial gluteal muscle proximally, and the middle gluteal muscle (arrowhead) can be seen immediately underneath the superficial gluteal muscle.

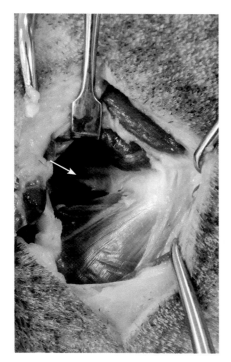

Figure 7. Proximal retraction of the middle gluteal muscle with a hand-held retractor. Note the insertion of the deep gluteal muscle at the base of the greater trochanter. The deep gluteal muscle (arrow) has a very characteristic orientation, with its fibres running in a cranioproximal direction from the greater trochanter of the femur.

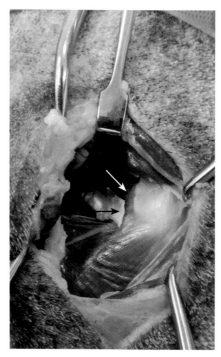

Figure 8. Tenotomy at the insertion of the deep gluteal muscle (black arrow). The tenotomy is done along one third to half of the width of the tendon, and the incision is then extended cranially in an L-shape through the deep gluteal muscle, parallel to the muscle fibres. The tenotomy is performed 1–2 mm cranial to the insertion of the tendon to allow resuturing during closure. The hip joint capsule (white arrow) is located immediately underneath the deep gluteal muscle.

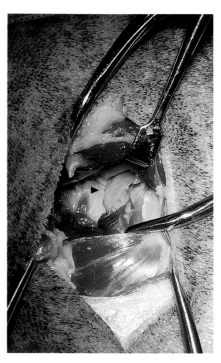

Figure 9. An incision has been made in the joint capsule (arrowhead) to allow exposure of the femoral head. An inverted T-shaped incision facilitates surgical closure of the joint capsule.

Exposure of the femoral head is achieved by externally rotating the limb while applying levering force to the femur, so that the patella is parallel to the floor and the cranial aspect of the patella is directed towards the ceiling (Fig. 10). If intact, the ligament of the head of the femur can be severed with a Hatt spoon (Figs. 11 and 12), thin curved scissors, or a small blade, to facilitate exposure of the femoral head and neck. A Hohmann retractor can also be used as a lever behind the femoral head or neck to expose the proximal femur.

Once the procedure is finished, the surgical site is copiously lavaged with sterile saline and closed in a standard fashion. A capsulorrhaphy is performed using monofilament absorbable or nonabsorbable suture material in an interrupted or continuous pattern. The author usually uses monofilament absorbable suture material, such as polydioxanone, in an interrupted (simple interrupted or cruciate) pattern (Fig. 13).

The tendon of the deep gluteal muscle is sutured to its origin on the greater trochanter of the femur with horizontal mattress sutures or a locking-loop pattern, before suturing the rest of the muscle with a simple continuous pattern. The author usually uses monofilament absorbable suture material (polydioxanone) for this purpose (Fig. 14).

In those cases in which the medial aspect of the vastus lateralis muscle has been disinserted, it must be sutured to the distal edge of the deep gluteal muscle. To do so, the author usually uses monofilament absorbable suture material (polydioxanone) in a simple continuous pattern. Retraction on the middle gluteal muscle is then released. Both leaves of the fascia lata are sutured to the cranial aspect of the biceps femoris muscle in a simple continuous pattern, and the tensor fasciae latae muscle is sutured to the superficial gluteal muscle using monofilament absorbable suture material (the author uses polydioxanone). Finally, the subcutaneous tissue is sutured in a simple continuous pattern with monofilament absorbable suture material, such as polyglecaprone 25, and the skin is apposed with monofilament nonabsorbable suture material (usually nylon suture in a simple interrupted or cruciate pattern), or using skin staples.

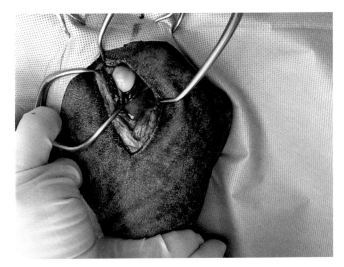

Figure 10. Exposure of the femoral head. The limb is externally rotated while applying mild levering force to the femur.

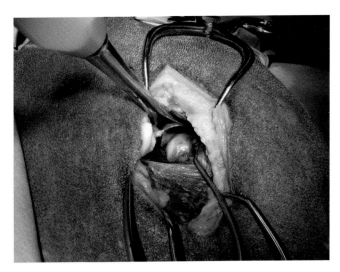

Figure 11. Exposure of the femoral head. If the round ligament is intact, it must be transected to allow adequate exposure. A Hatt spoon is placed around the femoral head.

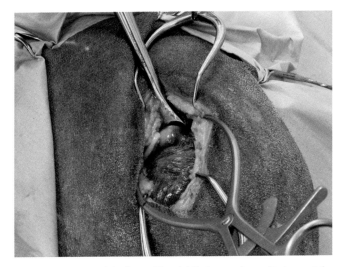

Figure 12. Exposure of the femoral head. A Hatt spoon is used to transect the round ligament. Once the round ligament is transected, the femoral head will easily luxate.

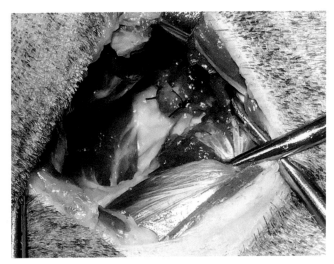

Figure 13. Close-up view of a capsulorraphy.

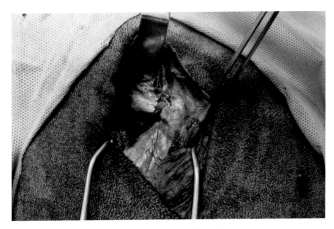

Figure 14. Resuturing of the deep gluteal muscle tendon.

HIP LUXATION

The hip joint has a ball and socket configuration, and its congruity and function are maintained by primary and secondary joint stabilisers (Wardlaw and McLaughlin, 2012). The main primary stabilisers of the hip are the ligament of the head of the femur, the joint capsule, and the dorsal acetabular rim. The main secondary stabilisers of the hip are the acetabular labrum (which ventrally forms the transverse acetabular ligament), the hydrostatic pressure created by the synovial fluid, and the periarticular muscles. For hip luxation to occur, there must be disruption of at least two of the primary stabilisers of the hip joint (Wardlaw and McLaughlin, 2012).

> Hip luxations are mostly traumatic in origin, but the amount of trauma required to cause luxation depends on whether there is an underlying hip pathology.

Animals with advanced hip dysplasia may suffer hip luxation following minimal trauma, while animals with normal hips require major trauma for luxation to occur.

Hip luxation is the most common joint luxation in the dog, accounting for 90 % of cases (Wardlaw and McLaughlin, 2012). It most commonly occurs in a craniodorsal direction, so that the head of the femur is located cranial and dorsal to the acetabulum; this accounts for approximately 75 % of hip luxations (Basher et al., 1986; DeCamp et al., 2016). Less commonly, luxation occurs in a caudoventral, caudodorsal or cranioventral direction.

The diagnosis of hip luxation is based on the patient's history, orthopaedic examination and diagnostic tests. As most cases are traumatic in nature, 50 % present with major concurrent injuries that need to be investigated and treated before addressing the hip luxation (DeCamp et al., 2016). Most of the time, the patient's owner has witnessed or is aware of a traumatic episode leading to hip luxation. The patient's history may also suggest previous hip pathology (history of stiffness or intermittent episodes of lameness) which could have contributed to luxation.

Patients with hip luxation are usually ambulatory, unless the luxation is bilateral or accompanied by other orthopaedic or neurological conditions. The clinical presentation is usually different depending on the direction of the hip luxation. Patients with a craniodorsal hip luxation are usually ambulatory, but frequently have a non-weight-bearing lameness, with the affected limb externally rotated, adducted and appearing shorter than the contralateral limb. The greater trochanter of the femur can be palpated in a more cranial and dorsal position when compared to that of the contralateral limb (in unilateral hip luxations). An increase in the distance between the greater trochanter of the femur and the ischial tuberosity will be noticeable in patients with craniodorsal hip luxation. A relatively easy way to diagnose a craniodorsal hip luxation is to perform the "thumb test". This test involves placing the thumb in the anatomical depression (ischiatic notch) between the greater trochanter of the femur and the ischial tuberosity, and externally rotating the femur at the same time. In normal animals, this manoeuvre will result in a displacement or compression of the finger between the greater trochanter and the ischium, while this will not occur in animals with craniodorsal hip luxation.

Patients with caudoventral hip luxation are clinically more severely affected and are almost always non-weight-bearing on the affected limb. In these patients, the limb is abducted, internally rotated and appears longer than the contralateral unaffected limb. Palpation of the hip area reveals a caudal and ventral displacement of the greater trochanter, which shortens the distance between the greater trochanter and the ischiatic tuberosity.

Regardless of the direction of the luxation, a pain response is elicited and crepitus is identified when the hip is manipulated through its range of motion.

Lateral and ventrodorsal radiographs are diagnostic in hip luxation (Figs. 15 and 16). They will indicate the direction of luxation and whether there are any concurrent injuries that may modify the treatment plan, such as hip dysplasia or fractures of the pelvis, femoral head, femoral neck and acetabulum (Figs. 17 and 18).

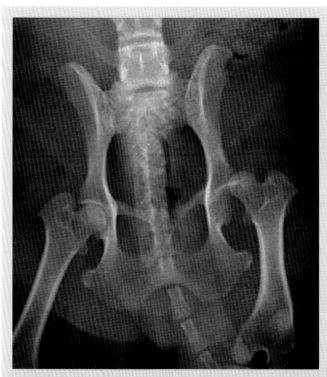

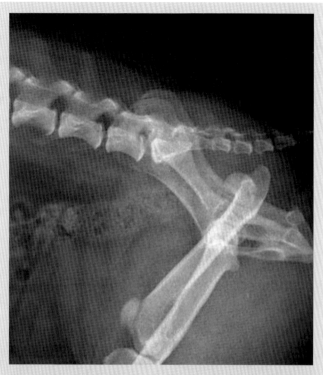

Figure 15. Ventrodorsal radiograph of the pelvis of a dog showing a left cranial hip luxation. There are no visible fractures affecting the pelvis or the proximal femur. The acetabulum is deep, with no evidence of osteoarthritis, and the femoral head has a normal shape.

Figure 16. Lateral radiograph of the pelvis of the same dog as in Fig. 15, showing a craniodorsal hip luxation. There are no visible fractures affecting the pelvis or the proximal femur.

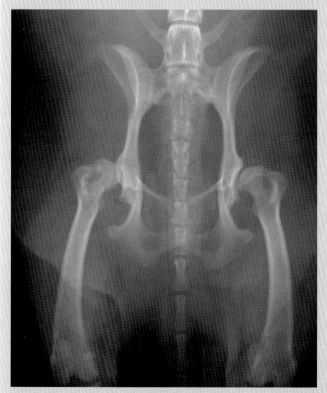

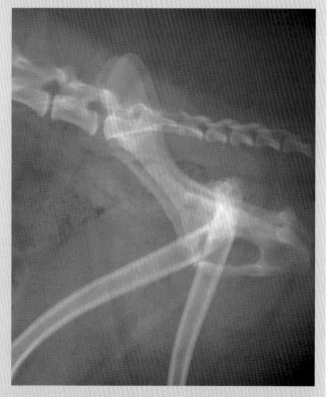

Figure 17. Ventrodorsal radiograph of the pelvis of a dog showing a right cranial hip luxation. This dog has severe signs of hip dysplasia, with remodelling of the acetabulum and the femoral head and neck. This patient has a concurrent left medial patellar luxation.

Figure 18. Lateral radiograph of the pelvis of the same dog as in Fig. 17 showing a craniodorsal hip luxation.

Hip luxations can be treated by closed or open reduction. Open reduction is more successful, with an average success rate of approximately 85 % (Fox, 1991; McLaughlin, 1995; Rochat, 2016). Other concurrent life-threatening injuries need to be prioritised but, if possible, the luxation should be reduced within the first 3–4 days. Chronic luxation results in articular cartilage damage due to friction of the femoral head against the pelvis, leading to pain and the likelihood of long-term degenerative joint disease once reduced. In chronic luxation, changes occur in the soft tissues around the acetabulum (joint capsule, remnants of the round ligament) which, combined with haematoma formation, can make closed reduction of the hip very challenging. There is also some degree of muscle contraction, which further complicates hip reduction and predisposes to reluxation. Therefore, the goal is to achieve hip reduction as soon as possible to prevent these changes and to apply some stabilising support. Stabilisation techniques (bandages and/or implants) aim to maintain hip reduction in the short and medium term while the soft tissues heal. In the long term, periarticular fibrosis is expected to maintain hip reduction (Douglas, 2000; Wardlaw and McLaughlin, 2012).

The following techniques are indicated in acute cases in which hip luxation is not related to hip dysplasia and there are no concurrent fractures of the femoral head or neck or the acetabulum. In those cases in which there are concurrent pathologies (significant hip dysplasia), abrasion of the articular cartilage, or nonreconstructable fractures of the acetabulum or femoral head and neck, salvage procedures should be considered, such as total hip replacement or femoral head and neck excision.

CLOSED REDUCTION

INTRODUCTION
This is a relatively simple procedure that does not require any specific equipment. It is very challenging to perform in a sedated patient, so general anaesthesia should be considered if the patient is stable.

INDICATIONS
Closed reduction of a hip luxation can be performed when there is an acute traumatic luxation with no radiographic evidence of significant hip dysplasia or concurrent hip fractures. This technique is more successful when performed during the first 3–4 days after hip luxation, before the development

of periarticular soft tissue changes and muscle contraction. It is advised to attempt this hip reduction method initially, as the risk of interfering with future open techniques if it is unsuccessful is relatively low (Bone et al., 1984; DeCamp et al., 2016). Closed hip reduction is also performed immediately before an open technique to facilitate the surgical approach to the hip.

SURGICAL PLANNING
Routine orthogonal pelvic radiographs are indicated to determine the direction of the hip luxation and rule out concurrent fractures or pre-existing hip conditions (hip dysplasia, Legg–Calvé–Perthes disease).

TECHNIQUE
The patient is positioned in lateral recumbency with the affected limb uppermost. For a craniodorsal luxation, the limb is externally rotated while applying traction in a caudodistal direction. An assistant should apply countertraction with soft, inelastic material (for example, a towel) placed around the patient's inguinal area. Once the femoral head is superimposed on the acetabulum, the limb is internally rotated and abducted while applying pressure on the greater trochanter to achieve hip reduction. A distinct "popping" sensation is usually felt when the femoral head reduces into the acetabulum.

In caudoventral luxations, the head of the femur is usually trapped inside the obturator foramen and needs to be disengaged. Applying traction and abduction on the limb as well as countertraction on the ischiatic tuberosity will enable the femoral head to disengage from the obturator foramen. If this is not sufficient, it may be useful to apply mild ventral force to the femoral head through rectal palpation while applying concurrent traction and abduction on the limb. Once the femoral head is freed from the obturator foramen, the femur is moved towards the acetabulum in a craniodorsal direction and the hip is reduced as previously described by abducting and internally rotating the limb while applying pressure on the greater trochanter.

The acetabulum is often filled with soft tissue (such as remnants of the joint capsule) and blood clots that prevent adequate hip reduction and predispose the patient to reluxation. Once the hip is reduced, in order to minimise the risk of reluxation, medially directed pressure is applied on the greater trochanter while moving the hip through various range of motion cycles. This manoeuvre will help to displace any soft tissues and achieve better reduction.

POSTOPERATIVE MANAGEMENT

It is recommended that an Ehmer sling is used to immobilise the reduced hip and thus minimise the likelihood of reluxation. An Ehmer sling flexes the hip, and abducts and internally rotates the femur. The sling is maintained for 10–14 days, and the bandage is inspected every 3 days until it is removed. Ehmer slings are contraindicated in caudoventral luxations; instead, hobbles should be used for 2–3 weeks to maintain hip reduction.

If not contraindicated, patients are prescribed non-steroidal anti-inflammatory drugs (NSAIDs) for 2 weeks until the bandage is removed. Exercise should be restricted for the first 2–3 months after hip reduction, as this is the time necessary for the soft tissue healing process to take place. Owners are asked to keep their dogs on strict cage rest for 3–4 weeks (or small room rest in larger patients), with very short (5 minutes) walks using a short lead and an abdominal sling 3–4 times daily. After this, the length of the controlled lead walks should gradually be increased over the following 4–6 weeks. After 8–10 weeks, very short periods (5 minutes initially) of off-lead exercise can be introduced at the end of each walk. The duration of unrestricted exercise should be progressively increased over a 3- to 4-week period.

OUTCOME

The prognosis is considered excellent when hip reduction is maintained. The outcome as assessed by owners was significantly better in patients treated by closed reduction than in patients treated by DeVita pinning, extracapsular suture stabilisation and femoral head and neck excision (Evers et al., 1997). Normal gait or mild long-term lameness has been reported in 84 % of cases (Bone et al., 1984), and in ventral luxations treated by closed reduction alone, 80 % of animals return to normal gait and limb function (Thacker and Schrader, 1985). The long-term prognosis will depend on the degree of damage to articular cartilage present on the femoral head and acetabulum. Attempting hip reduction several times can lead to articular damage and subsequent long-term osteoarthritis. Therefore, an open reduction technique should be performed if the hip reluxates easily after reduction, if reduction attempts are unsuccessful, or if the femoral head can be felt rubbing excessively against the acetabulum during reduction attempts.

COMPLICATIONS

The most common complication after a closed reduction technique is hip reluxation, as reported in approximately 50–65 % of patients (Bone et al., 1984; Basher et al., 1986). Reluxation occurs most frequently during the first 3 weeks after hip reduction.

Another complication of closed reduction is further damage to the articular cartilage during reduction attempts. Bandage-associated complications such as skin wounds or bandage slipping are common.

HIP TOGGLE

INTRODUCTION

Hip toggle stabilisation is a commonly used technique to stabilise the hip joint, and was first described by Knowles et al. (1953). With this technique, the ruptured ligament of the head of the femur is replaced with synthetic material that provides initial stability while the soft tissues heal and peri–articular fibrosis forms (DeCamp et al., 2016).

> The aim of the hip toggle technique is to mimic the functions of the ligament of the head of the femur, by maintaining hip reduction in the short to medium term while allowing a good range of motion in the hip and early weight-bearing on the affected limb.

A hip toggle system relies on the mechanical properties of its components. The surgical implants need to resist the forces that are generated in the hip during weight-bearing and over its range of motion. A hip toggle system involves a toggle component (either a toggle rod or a toggle pin) with associated suture material. The biomechanical properties of different toggle configurations and suture materials have been investigated, and at the time of writing, it is difficult to determine which is the best implant for hip toggle stabilisation. Although it has been shown that both toggle rods and toggle pins can be used in hip toggle constructs, it has been suggested that toggle rods might be more suitable and that toggle failure is more common with home-made toggle pins (Baltzer et al., 2001; Demko et al., 2006; Jha and Kowaleski, 2012). For this reason, it is recommended to use commercially available toggle rods to avoid individual variations that might occur when creating home-made toggle pins. An in vitro biomechanical study using home-made toggle pins showed a 60 % incidence of deformity or breakage of the toggle (Flynn et al., 1994). Therefore, home-made toggles are no longer recommended (Wardlaw and McLaughlin, 2012). A variety of suture materials have been used in hip toggles in an attempt to reduce implant failure and subsequent hip reluxation. Suture materials include monofilament nylon, braided polyester, woven polyester and braided polyblends. Guidelines regarding appropriate implant size have been proposed (Rochat, 2016), with a 2.7 mm-diameter toggle system being recommended for patients weighing less than 5 kg, a 3.2 mm-diameter toggle system for animals weighing 6–30 kg, and a 4 mm-diameter toggle system for animals weighing more than 30 kg. The successful use of 3.2 mm toggle rods in cats with a mean weight of 4.3 kg has also been reported, and although the size of the toggle rod reduced the pelvic canal diameter by 16.2 %, it did not have any clinical consequences (Pratesi et al., 2012).

INDICATIONS

This technique is indicated when stable hip reduction cannot be achieved using a closed technique, or when hip reluxation occurs following closed reduction. It is used in acute or chronic cases of traumatic hip luxation, when there are no signs of significant hip dysplasia and no concurrent fractures of the acetabulum or of the femoral head or neck. Hip toggle stabilisation is used as the first line of treatment when early postoperative weight-bearing is desired, for example in patients that will not tolerate a non-weight-bearing bandage or when other limbs are injured.

SURGICAL PLANNING

Routine orthogonal pelvic radiographs are indicated to determine the direction of the hip luxation and rule out concurrent fractures or pre-existing hip conditions (hip dysplasia, Legg–Calvé–Perthes disease).

SURGICAL TECHNIQUE

A standard craniolateral approach to the hip is made as previously described. Careful examination of the joint capsule, articular cartilage, and anatomy of the acetabulum and femoral head is mandatory (Fig. 19). Any soft tissue or blood clots should be removed from the acetabulum to allow proper hip reduction. The remnants of the ruptured ligament of the head of the femur should also be excised. When possible, it is important to preserve the remnants of the joint capsule as capsulorrhaphy will provide further stability to the hip toggle technique.

A hole is drilled that penetrates through the acetabulum at the level of the acetabular fossa (Figs. 20 and 21), taking

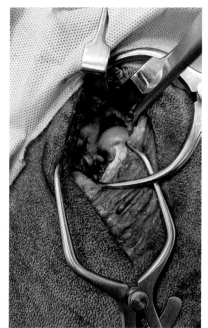

Figure 19. Exposure of the acetabulum and femoral head. Careful examination of the joint capsule, articular cartilage, acetabulum, and femoral head is mandatory before performing a hip toggle procedure.

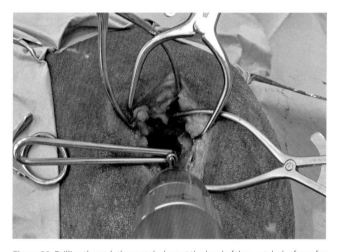

Figure 20. Drilling through the acetabulum at the level of the acetabular fossa for hip toggle positioning. Extreme care must be taken not to perforate the rectum. A drill guide is used to protect the soft tissues and femoral head.

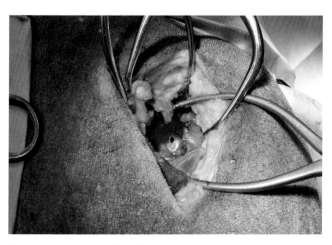

Figure 21. Close-up view of the drilled hole in the acetabulum.

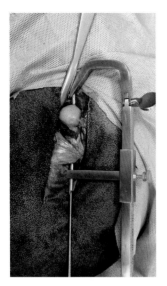

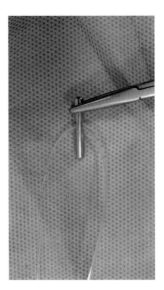

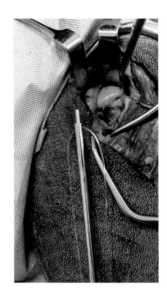

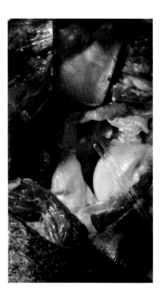

Figure 22. Positioning of a C-shaped guide to drill a tunnel from the lateral aspect of the femur (at the level of the third trochanter) through the femoral neck to the fovea capitis. This tunnel may be drilled in either a normograde or a retrograde fashion.

Figure 23. Hip toggle rod system. The toggle rod is held with needle holders, and a monofilament nylon suture passes through the toggle rod.

Figure 24. Hip toggle introducer with the toggle rod inserted at the end. A hip toggle introducer can be very helpful to pass the toggle through the acetabular hole.

Figure 25. Insertion of the toggle rod with attached suture material through the hole previously drilled in the acetabular fossa. Pulling each end of the suture alternately allows the toggle to be placed flat against the medial aspect of the acetabular wall.

extreme care not to perforate the rectum. A drill sleeve should be used to protect the femoral head and surrounding soft tissues. The diameter of hole must be slightly larger than that of the combination of toggle and suture material to allow easy insertion. As a guideline, a 2.7 mm drill bit is used in cats and small-breed dogs (standard 2.0 mm toggles), a 3.5 mm drill bit is used in medium-breed dogs (standard 3.0 to 3.2 mm toggles), and 4.5 mm drill bit is used in large-breed dogs (standard 4.0 mm toggle). However, the acetabular hole can be enlarged if needed to allow easy insertion of the toggle together with the selected suture material.

A tunnel is then drilled from the fovea capitis of the femoral head through the femoral neck to the lateral aspect of the femur at the level of the third trochanter (Fig. 22). The tunnel should be wide enough to contain both suture strands; its diameter will depend on the patient's size and the material used. As a guideline, a 2.0 mm drill bit is used in cats and small-breed dogs, a 2.5 mm drill bit in medium-size dogs, and a 3.5 mm drill bit in giant-breed dogs. A C-shaped guide allows precise drilling of this tunnel.

A toggle rod with attached suture material (Figs. 23 and 24) is inserted through the hole drilled in the acetabular fossa, and placed flat against the medial aspect of the acetabular wall by pulling each end of the suture alternately (Fig. 25). This locks the toggle medial to the acetabular wall.

The ends of the suture material are passed through the tunnel previously created in the femoral neck, to exit on the lateral aspect of the femur. A suture passer is needed when using braided polyblend material, but monofilament nylon can be driven through the tunnel without a suture passer. Once the hip is reduced, the sutures can be secured on the lateral aspect of the femur in two ways. They can be tightened over an implant such as a sterile button or another toggle rod provided in commercial kits (Fig. 26), or an alternative is to drill a new tunnel in the lateral femoral cortex in a caudocranial direction (immediately proximal to the level of exit of the sutures in the lateral femoral cortex), pass one strand of the suture through it, and tie or crimp the strand to the other strand (Figs. 27, 28 and 29).

Another factor to take into consideration is the type of suture material used. A surgeon's knot with 6–8 throws (Rochat, 2016) should be used to tighten the suture; however, when using monofilament nylon, it is very challenging to obtain a secure surgeon's knot and a metallic crimp tube can be used instead. The suture must be tight enough to prevent subluxation, but it must also allow a full range of motion of the hip.

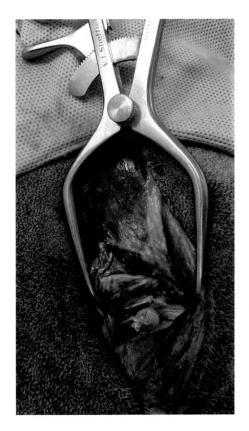

◀ Figure 26. The sutures can be secured by tightening them to a sterile button on the lateral aspect of the femur using a surgeon's knot with 6–8 throws.

▼ Figure 27. A tunnel has been drilled in the lateral femoral cortex in a caudocranial direction (immediately proximal to the exit of the sutures in the lateral femoral cortex). A suture thread has been passed through this tunnel.

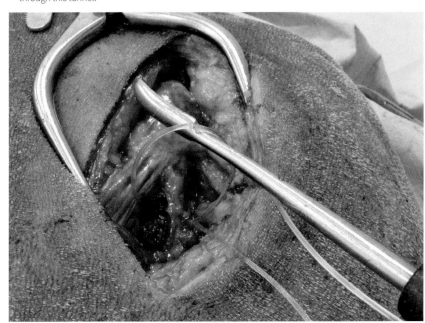

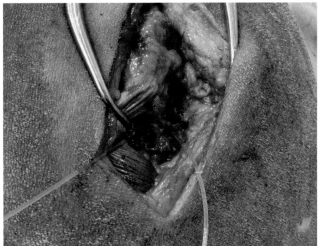

Figure 28. One strand of the suture has been passed through the newly drilled femoral tunnel.

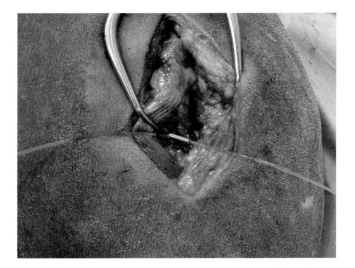

Figure 29. A crimp tube has been used to secure the suture on the lateral aspect of the femur.

POSTOPERATIVE MANAGEMENT

Postoperative radiographs are indicated to assess hip reduction and implant positioning (Figs. 30 and 31). Patients are expected to bear weight immediately after surgery, and no bandaging support is needed.

If not contraindicated, patients are prescribed NSAIDs for 2–3 weeks. Exercise is restricted for the first 2–3 months after surgery as this is the time necessary for the soft tissue healing process to take place. Owners are asked to keep their pets on strict cage rest for 3–4 weeks (or small room rest for large patients), with very short (5 minutes) walks using a short lead and an abdominal sling 3–4 times daily. Gentle physiotherapy may be performed during these first 4 weeks. It is then recommended to gradually increase the length of the controlled lead walks for the following 4 weeks and to introduce controlled hydrotherapy. The author performs a

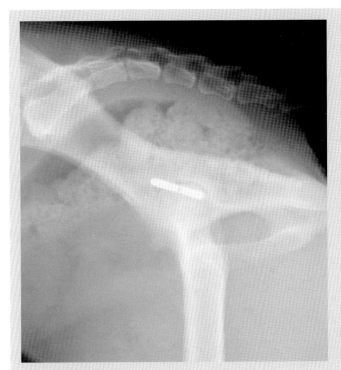

Figure 30. Postoperative lateral radiograph after a hip toggle procedure showing adequate hip reduction and good implant positioning.

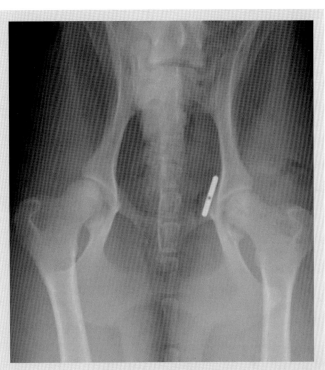

Figure 31. Postoperative ventrodorsal radiograph after a hip toggle procedure showing adequate hip reduction and good implant positioning.

radiographic assessment of the hip and implants 6–8 weeks after the procedure, or sooner if there is any deterioration in the patient's gait. After 8 weeks, very short periods (5 minutes initially) of off-lead exercise can be introduced at the end of each walk. The duration of unrestricted exercise should progressively be increased over a 3–4 week period, after which the patient can return to normal activity.

OUTCOME

This technique has a very good functional outcome both in dogs (Demko, 2006; Ash et al., 2012; Kieves et al., 2014) and cats (Ash et al., 2012; Pratesi et al., 2012). A recent report on the use of this technique in nine patients (toy breeds and cats) showed that only one patient had mild residual lameness (Ash et al., 2012). When assessed by owner questionnaire, the long-term overall quality of life of 14 cats following this procedure was reported as excellent in 91 % and very good in 8 % of the cases (Pratesi et al., 2012). Of these cats, 64 % were considered to have normal limb function, while 9 % of the owners considered that the final outcome interfered frequently with the activity or behaviour of their cat. Another study in 17 dogs reported the long-term limb function to be good (12 %) or excellent (88 %) with all patients considered pain free (Kieves et al., 2014). Gait analysis was

performed in 6 of these 17 dogs and results showed an equal use of both hindlimbs. Finally, radiographic assessment of six of the patients a mean of 7.5 months after the procedure showed no progression of osteoarthritis in the operated joint (Kieves et al., 2014). Another study of 62 cases indicated that, when assessed by their owners, 85 % of the patients were sound or had a minimal degree of lameness (Demko et al., 2006).

COMPLICATIONS

Complications include premature implant failure (suture or toggle breakage) leading to reluxation, fractures of the femoral head or neck, rectal perforation, articular cartilage damage, surgery-related infections, and sciatic neuropraxia.

The most common complication after hip toggle surgery is recurrence of hip luxation. Traditionally, reluxation rates have been reported to be between 11 and 25 % (Duff and Bennett, 1982; Bone et al., 1984; Flynn et al., 1994). A reluxation rate of 14 % was reported with hip toggles when using polydioxanone as the suture material in cats (Pratesi et al., 2012). In this study, capsulorrhaphy could not be performed in 93 % of the cats due to severe damage to the joint capsule. More recently, there has been an increased interest in new suture materials with superior biomechanical properties and commercially available toggle rods in an attempt to reduce reluxation rates. A reluxation rate of 11 % has been reported when using monofilament nylon and polyester suture material (Demko et al., 2006), while the reported long-term reluxation rate when using braided polyblend material is 5.8 % (Kieves et al., 2014). However, the biomechanical advantages of the new braided suture materials should be weighed against the potential complications of multifilament sutures, such as local tissue reaction and risk of implant-related infections.

ILIOFEMORAL SUTURE

INTRODUCTION

Placement of an iliofemoral suture is a relatively simple technique. An initial description of this technique, which involved placing sutures between the psoas minor and the middle gluteal muscles, was documented in 1988 and showed encouraging long-term results in 11 patients (Mehl, 1988). The technique as performed nowadays was described in 1992, and used multifilament nonabsorbable suture material in 14 dogs and 3 cats with excellent results (Meij et al., 1992). A variation of the technique has been reported, in which the iliac suture is placed through the insertion of the rectus femoris muscle rather than through an iliac bone tunnel (Shani et al., 2004). The iliofemoral suture mimics the effect of an Ehmer sling and limits the range of motion of the hip. As with any synthetic suture, the iliofemoral suture will eventually fail by loosening or breaking.

> The function of the iliofemoral suture is to provide hip stability during the first weeks after hip reduction, while in the long term, hip reduction is maintained by healed soft tissues and periarticular fibrosis.

Both monofilament (Shani et al., 2004) and multifilament (Martini et al., 2001) sutures have been used for this procedure. The author routinely uses monofilament nylon in this procedure as good outcomes have been reported using this material (Shani et al., 2004) and the risk of postoperative infection is lower than when using multifilament material. He also uses metallic crimp tubes instead of knots to secure the suture.

INDICATIONS

This surgery is indicated for the treatment of acute or chronic craniodorsal hip luxation, although it has also been used sporadically in ventral hip luxation (Meij et al., 1992; Martini et al., 2001). This technique is indicated when stable hip reduction cannot be achieved using a closed technique, or when hip reluxation occurs following closed reduction. It is used when there are no signs of significant hip dysplasia and no concurrent fractures of the acetabulum or of the femoral head or neck. The technique allows early postoperative weight-bearing.

SURGICAL PLANNING

Routine orthogonal pelvic radiographs are indicated to determine the direction of luxation and rule out concurrent fractures or pre-existing hip conditions (hip dysplasia, Legg–Calvé–Perthes disease).

SURGICAL TECHNIQUE

A standard craniolateral approach to the hip joint is recommended. Hip assessment and reduction is carried out as previously described. If possible, capsulorrhaphy should be performed.

A 1.5 to 2.0 mm hole (slightly larger than the diameter of the suture material used) is drilled at the site of insertion of the rectus femoris in the ilium (on the ventral aspect of the ilium, cranial to the acetabulum) in a lateral to medial direction (Fig. 32).

A suture thread is passed through the hole in the ilium in a lateral to medial direction. The suture end is retrieved from the medial aspect of the ilium using curved haemostat forceps placed under the ventral aspect of the ilium (Figs. 33 and 34).

Another hole is drilled in the femur in a caudocranial direction at the base of the greater trochanter (Fig. 35).

Using straight haemostat forceps, one suture end is passed in a craniocaudal direction underneath the insertion of the gluteal muscles on the greater trochanter (Fig. 36). It is then brought back in a caudocranial direction through the femoral hole, creating a figure-of-eight pattern (Fig. 37 and 38).

The hip joint is reduced, the femur is slightly internally rotated and abducted and the ends of the suture are secured together with knots or crimps (Figs. 39 and 40). Closure of the surgical site is standard as previously described.

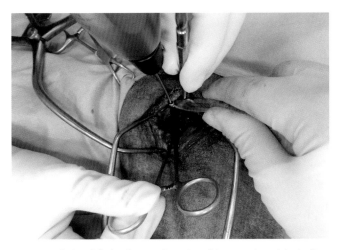

Figure 32. A hole is drilled at the site of insertion of the rectus femoris in the ilium in a lateral to medial direction.

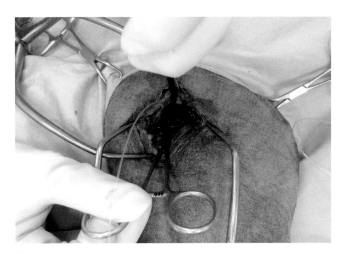

Figure 33. A suture is passed through the hole in the ilium in a lateral to medial direction, and retrieved using curved haemostat forceps under the ventral aspect of the ilium.

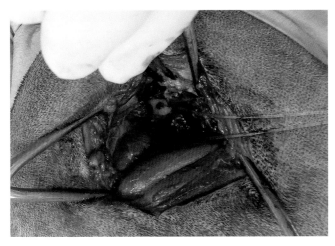

Figure 34. The suture has been passed and retrieved through a hole in the ventral aspect of the ilium, at the site of insertion of the rectus femoris muscle.

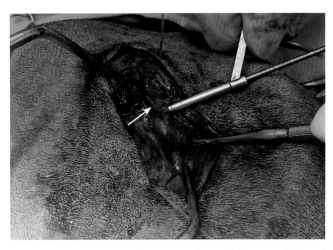

Figure 35. A hole is drilled in the femur in a caudocranial direction at the base of the greater trochanter (arrow).

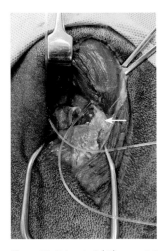

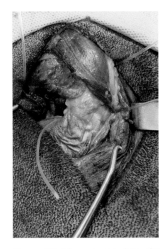

Figure 36. Using straight haemostat forceps, one suture end is passed in a craniocaudal direction underneath the insertion of the gluteal muscles in the greater trochanter (arrow).

Figure 37. The suture is brought back in a caudocranial direction through the previously drilled hole at the base of the greater trochanter.

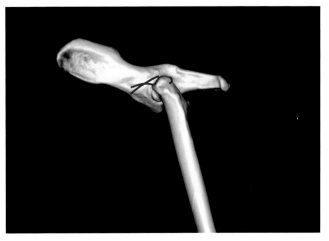

Figure 38. CT scan reconstruction of a pelvis indicating the pathway followed by the iliofemoral suture to create the figure-of-eight pattern.

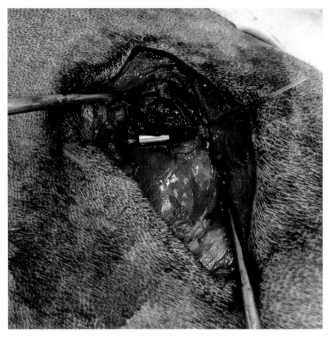

Figure 39. Positioning of the suture and crimp tube before securing the suture.

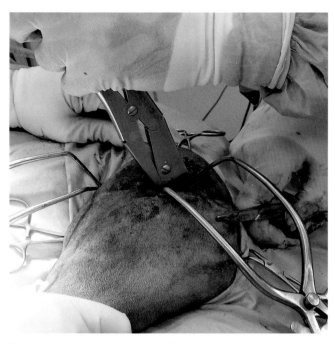

Figure 40. The sutures are moderately tightened and crimped. Caution must be taken not to overtighten the sutures.

POSTOPERATIVE MANAGEMENT

Postoperative radiographs are indicated to assess hip reduction and implant positioning (Figs. 41 and 42). Although the use of a postoperative bandage has been described, several reports do not support this practice and it is therefore not recommended (Martini et al., 2001; Shani et al., 2004).

Postoperative management after an iliofemoral suture is very similar to that following a hip toggle procedure. If not contraindicated, patients are prescribed NSAIDs for 2–3 weeks. Exercise should be restricted during the first 2–3 months after surgery as this is the time necessary for the soft tissue healing process to take place. Owners are asked to keep their dog on strict cage rest for 3–4 weeks (or small room rest in large patients) with very short (5 minutes) walks 3–4 times daily. These walks should be at a slow pace, using a short lead and an abdominal sling. Gentle physiotherapy

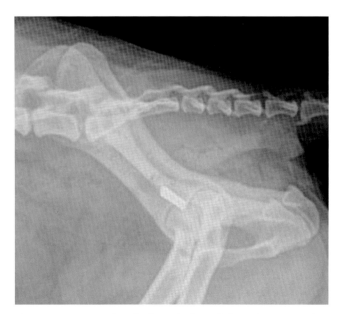

Figure 41. Postoperative lateral radiograph after an iliofemoral suture procedure showing adequate hip reduction and good implant positioning.

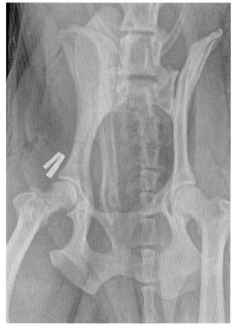

Figure 42. Postoperative ventrodorsal radiograph after an iliofemoral suture procedure showing adequate hip reduction and good implant positioning.

can be performed during the first 4 weeks. The length of the controlled lead walks can then be gradually increased for the following 4 weeks. Controlled hydrotherapy is also recommended. After 8 weeks, very short periods (5 minutes initially) off the lead can be introduced at the end of the walks. The duration of unrestricted exercise can then be increased progressively over a 3–4 week period, after which the patient can return to unrestricted exercise.

OUTCOME

The reported outcome in patients that have undergone this technique is very good. Animals should bear weight within 10 days of surgery, and lameness should resolve within 30 days (Martini et al., 2001; Shani et al., 2004). In a study by Meij et al., 81 % of the patients were sound at follow-up appointments, and the outcome of the surgery was scored by their owners as excellent (Meij et al., 1992). The latest reports described no lameness or pain on manipulation of the hip over its range of motion at long-term follow-up, although in one study 4 out of 14 dogs had occasional lameness after vigorous exercise (Martini et al., 2001).

COMPLICATIONS

Potential complications of this technique include early implant failure leading to hip reluxation, iliac or trochanteric fractures, and surgery-related infections. No complications were seen in the most recent studies (Martini et al., 2001; Shani et al., 2004). A postoperative bandage was not used in any of these studies.

TRANSARTICULAR PIN

INTRODUCTION

Transarticular pinning was first described in 1980 (Bennet and Duff, 1980). It can be done both as an open and as a closed procedure. A Steinman pin or Kirschner wire (1.6–3.2 mm) is used to provide short-term stabilisation of the hip joint while the soft tissues heal and periarticular fibrosis develops, which will maintain hip reduction in the long term. While in place, the transarticular pin only allows hip flexion and extension. The relatively high complication rate compared with other techniques and the need to remove the implant after 2–3 weeks has made this technique less common than those already described.

INDICATIONS

> Transarticular pinning is indicated when a stable hip reduction cannot be achieved using a closed technique, or when hip reluxation occurs following closed reduction.

It is most commonly used in acute cases of traumatic hip luxation, when there are no signs of significant hip dysplasia and no concurrent fractures of the acetabulum or of the femoral head or neck. The technique is mainly used in small dogs and cats, as animals over 20 kg have a higher complication rate (Hunt and Henry, 1985).

SURGICAL PLANNING

Routine orthogonal pelvic radiographs are indicated to determine the direction of luxation and rule out concurrent fractures or pre-existing hip conditions (hip dysplasia, Legg–Calvé–Perthes disease).

SURGICAL TECHNIQUE

When used as a closed technique, the hip is first reduced and the limb is slightly abducted and internally rotated. The pin is inserted slightly distal to the base of the greater trochanter, and driven in a normograde direction through the femoral neck. The pin should exit at the fovea capitis of the femoral head and penetrate through the acetabulum a few millimetres into the pelvic canal.

Alternatively, if an open approach is used, the pin can be inserted in a normograde (Fig. 43) or retrograde direction. In a retrograde fashion, the pin is inserted from the fovea capitis (Fig. 44) through the femoral neck, aiming at the lateral aspect of the femur, distal to the base of the greater trochanter (Fig. 45). The pin is advanced until it protrudes 3–4 cm from the lateral aspect of the femur. The pin is then pulled from the lateral aspect of the femur (Fig. 46) until its tip is no longer visible at the fovea capitis. Once the hip is reduced, slight abduction and internal rotation are applied and the pin is advanced (Fig. 47) to penetrate a few millimetres into the acetabular wall as previously described.

When selecting the size of the pin, the author follows the guidelines by Rochat (2016) and uses a 1.6 mm Kirschner wire in animals weighing less than 7 kg. The size of the Steinman pin is progressively increased up to 2.4 mm in animals weighing less than 30 kg, and a 3.2 mm pin is used in animals weighing more than 30 kg. The pin should penetrate

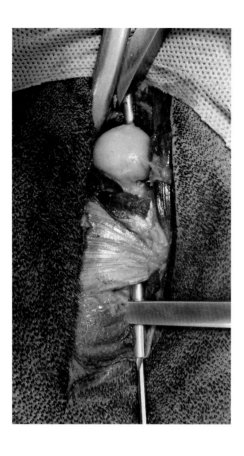

◀ Figure 43. Transarticular pin placement in a normograde fashion. A C-shaped guide has been used to drill a tunnel from the lateral aspect of the femur (at the level of the third trochanter) through the femoral neck to the fovea capitis.

▼ Figure 44. Transarticular pin placed in a retrograde fashion. The pin is inserted at the fovea capitis, passed through the femoral neck and exits on the lateral aspect of the femur (at the level of the third trochanter).

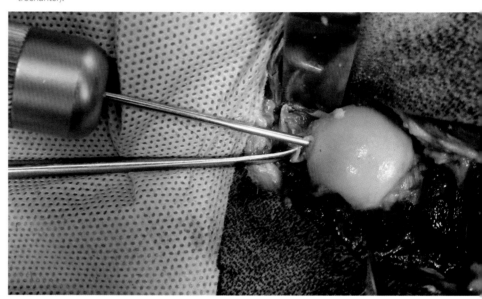

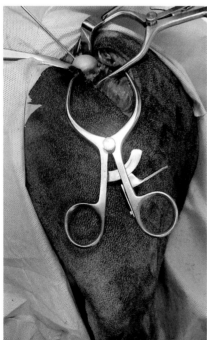

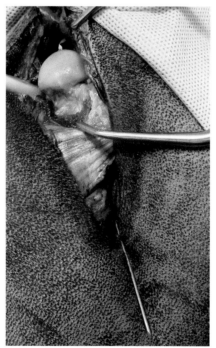

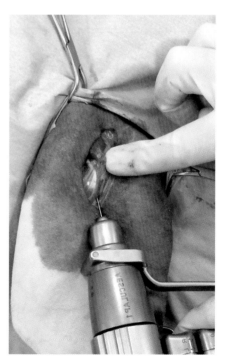

Figure 45. Transarticular pin placement in a retrograde fashion. The limb is externally rotated to allow pin placement in an adequate direction.

Figure 46. The pin is pulled from the lateral aspect of the femur until the tip is no longer visible at the fovea capitis. In this image, the pin needs to be pulled a few more millimetres before the hip is reduced.

Figure 47. Once the hip is reduced, slight abduction and internal rotation are applied and the pin is advanced to penetrate a few millimetres through the acetabular wall into the pelvic canal. The surgeon is pointing at the greater trochanter of the femur.

just a few millimetres (approximately 2–4 mm) beyond the acetabular wall to avoid rectal perforation. Predrilling the femoral neck tunnel with a smaller drill bit has been recommended to avoid femoral osteonecrosis (McCartney et al., 2011). A nonscrubbed assistant can assess the depth of pin penetration beyond the acetabular wall by rectal palpation. Once the pin is placed, it can be bent and cut short on the lateral aspect of the femur to avoid pin migration and minimise soft tissue irritation. Closure of the surgical site is as previously described.

POSTOPERATIVE MANAGEMENT

Postoperative radiographs are indicated to assess hip reduction and implant positioning (Figs. 48 and 49). Although not commonly needed, this stabilisation can be supported by an Ehmer sling for 10–12 days. The author does not use postoperative bandages on a routine basis, and removes the transarticular pin approximately 3 weeks after surgery.

If not contraindicated, patients are initially prescribed NSAIDs for 2–3 weeks; the duration of treatment should then be prolonged or resumed for 1 week after pin removal, which is done 2–3 weeks after the initial surgery. Exercise should be restricted during the first 2–3 months after surgery as this is the time necessary for the soft tissue healing process to take place. Owners are asked to keep their dogs on strict cage rest for 3–4 weeks (or small room rest in large patients), with very short (5 minutes) walks using a short lead and an abdominal sling 3–4 times daily. Gentle physiotherapy can be performed during the first 4 weeks. The author performs a radiographic assessment of the hip and implant 3 weeks after the procedure, and removes the transarticular pin at that time. It is then recommended to gradually increase the length of the controlled lead walks for the following 4 weeks and to introduce controlled hydrotherapy. After these first 8 weeks, very short periods (5 minutes initially) off the lead can be introduced at the end of the walks. Their duration should then be increased progressively over a 3–4 week period, after which the patient can return to unrestricted exercise.

Postoperative management of cats is more challenging. Strict cage rest combined with gentle physiotherapy is recommended for the first 6 weeks. After this initial period, room rest is advised for another 4 weeks, after which the patient can return to unrestricted exercise.

OUTCOME

The outcome of this technique is considered very good in 80 % of patients when combined with a postoperative Ehmer

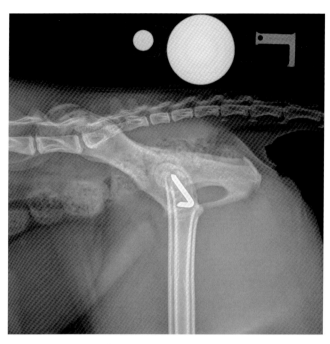

Figure 48. Postoperative lateral radiograph after a transarticular pin procedure, showing adequate hip reduction and good implant positioning.

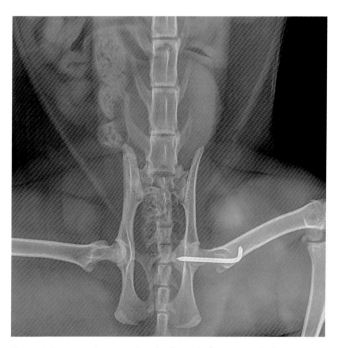

Figure 49. Postoperative ventrodorsal radiograph after a transarticular pin procedure showing adequate hip reduction and good implant positioning.

sling, although the success rate goes down to approximately 60 % in animals over 20 kg (Hunt and Henry, 1985). In another recent study using owner-based questionnaires, although 96 % of the owners were satisfied with the outcome of this procedure, 66 % of the dogs continued to have intermittent lameness or stiffness (McCartney et al., 2011). A study in 20 cats showed mild or no long-term osteoarthritis in 61 % of the cases, with 45 %, 35 % and 20 % of the owners reporting an excellent, very good, or good outcome respectively (Sissener et al., 2009). When assessed by a veterinary surgeon, the outcome was reported as excellent in 31 %, very good in 54 % and good in 15 % of the cats. The overall success rate in this study once complications were taken into account was 77 %. No postoperative sling was used in these cats.

COMPLICATIONS

Complications of this surgical technique include pin migration, pin breakage, pin bending, sciatic neuropraxia, surgery-related infections, and rectal perforation. Transarticular pinning can also damage the articular cartilage, which leads to osteoarthritis (Meij et al., 1992).

A 40 % incidence of pin breakage with a 14 % incidence of hip subluxation and a 7 % incidence of osteonecrosis and femoral head resorption has been reported in dogs (Hunt and Henry, 1985). A study assessing the outcome of 70 dogs with hip luxation treated using transarticular pinning revealed major complications in four dogs (5.7 %), including one dog with sciatic nerve damage, one dog with osteonecrosis, one dog with reluxation after pin removal and one dog with pin breakage (McCartney et al., 2011). In this same study, 45 % of the patients had swelling and discharge at the pin site while 7 % developed skin ulcers at the pin site. The overall outcome was classified as excellent in 23 cases, good in 41 cases, and poor in 4 cases. The technique failed in 2 out of the 70 cases.

Complications in this procedure seem to be related to the size of the animal. In a study of 20 cats treated using transarticular pinning, one case of pin bending occurred (a 1.2 mm pin was used), while 15 % of the patients had hip reluxation after removal of the transarticular pin, and 8 % of the patients had complete femoral head resorption (Sissener et al., 2009). No pin breakage was found in this study.

HIP DYSPLASIA

Hip dysplasia is one of the most common reasons for hindlimb lameness in dogs, and the main cause of hip osteoarthritis (Smith et al., 2012). The exact cause of hip dysplasia is unknown, but it is suspected to be multifactorial, with a combination of genetic predisposition and environmental contributing factors.

> Hip laxity is a major initiating cause for hip dysplasia.

Congruity of the hip through its range of motion is affected by hip laxity, which creates an inflammatory process in the hip joint and wear of the articular cartilage due to abnormal force distribution through the joint and abnormal contact between the acetabulum and femoral head. These changes lead to osteoarthritis (Smith et al., 2012).

Although hip dysplasia can occur in any dog, it is more commonly reported in large breeds (Smith et al., 2012). Hip dysplasia is mainly seen in two groups: young animals (4–12 months), in which clinical signs are due to hip laxity; and animals older than 15 months, in which the disease is chronic and the clinical signs are more likely to be associated with the development of osteoarthritis (DeCamp et al., 2016).

The clinical signs are very variable. Typically, animals present with acute or chronic hindlimb lameness with short strides. Patients with bilateral hip dysplasia may show a classic swaying gait. Lameness may be unilateral or bilateral. Clinically affected patients often have difficulty standing up or jumping, are reluctant to exercise, and run with a "bunny-hopping" gait. Sometimes, the owners describe a "clicking" noise when the patient is walking or running, which is due to the subluxation and reduction that takes place in very lax hips. Clinical signs in chronic cases tend to be more subtle and progress more slowly, while younger patients can have acute episodes of lameness. Caution must be taken when an adult patient with ongoing chronic hip dysplasia presents with an acute severe episode of lameness, as this acute deterioration is often due to a concurrent pathology (such as cranial cruciate ligament disease).

A complete general physical, orthopaedic and neurological examination is recommended in all patients. On orthopaedic examination, patients with hip dysplasia may show discomfort or pain on manipulation of the hip, crepitus as the hip is manipulated through its range of motion and altered stance positions with a wide or narrow stance (Smith et al., 2012). In more chronic cases, a decreased hip range of motion may be observed, particularly in extension. The degree of muscle waste on the affected limb depends on the chronicity and severity of the clinical signs. Sometimes, an increase in the forelimb muscle mass might be seen due to chronic weight shifting from the hindlimbs (these dogs will show bilateral tarsal hyperextension when shifting the weight to the forelimbs). A positive Barden or Ortolani/Barlow test is used to confirm hip laxity, which is more common in young animals. These tests are preferably done with the patient under general anaesthesia.

Hip dysplasia is diagnosed based on physical examination and radiographs (Figs. 50 and 51). Young patients with mild hip dysplasia might not develop radiographic signs until they are adults. Therefore, it is recommended to wait until the patient is 2 years old to make a radiographic diagnosis of hip dysplasia in mild cases, as it has been shown that the diagnosis is 92–95 % accurate at that age (Jessen and Spurrell, 1972). Typically, the extended ventrodorsal radiographic view is used to assess the congruity between the femoral head and the acetabulum at the cranial acetabular margin, the femoral head coverage by the dorsal acetabular rim (a normal hip has more than 50 % coverage), the acetabular depth and shape, the femoral head shape, and the presence of osteophytosis (e.g. caudolateral curvilinear and/or circumferential femoral head osteophytes). Measuring the Norberg angle has been used to diagnose hip subluxation (Fig. 52). Traditionally, a Norberg angle of less than 105 degrees was considered diagnostic of hip subluxation. However, this has recently been challenged and breed-specific angles have been suggested (Culp et al., 2006). Radiographs of young animals with hip laxity may show no changes. Distraction techniques were developed to measure passive hip laxity, using the PennHIP® score to differentiate normal dogs (distraction index below 0.3) from dogs with hip laxity (distraction index of at least 0.3).

Conservative treatment of hip dysplasia is based on exercise control, physical rehabilitation therapy (physiotherapy and hydrotherapy), weight management and pain relief medication (most frequently NSAIDs). Other treatments include polysulfated glycosaminoglycan and oral nutritional supplements such as omega-3 fatty acids.

The surgical treatment of hip dysplasia varies depending on the age of the patient, the degree of hip subluxation and

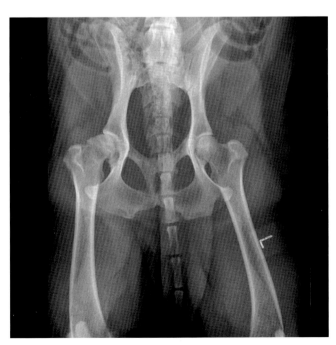

Figure 50. Ventrodorsal radiograph of a dog with right hip dysplasia. There is coxofemoral subluxation with severe osteoarthritic changes at the femoral head and thickening of the femoral neck. Poor coverage of the femoral head by the dorsal acetabular rim is also observed. The left hip is normal.

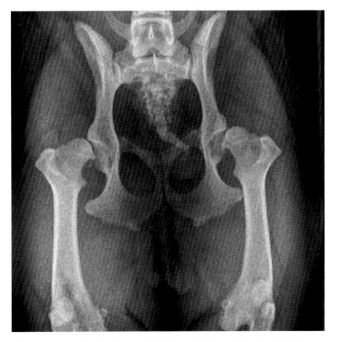

Figure 51. Ventrodorsal radiograph of a dog with bilateral hip dysplasia. There is bilateral severe coxofemoral subluxation with remodelling of the right acetabulum and of the femoral head and neck bilaterally.

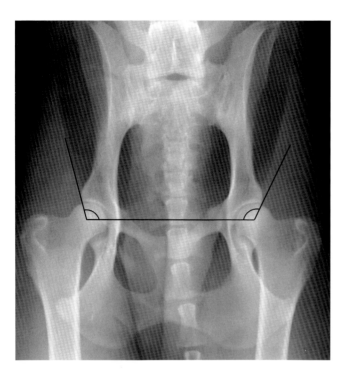

Figure 52. Ventrodorsal radiograph of a dog with a normal hip. To calculate the Norberg angle, a line is drawn between the geometric centres of the femoral heads. A second line is drawn between the centre of each femoral head and the craniolateral aspect of the acetabular rim. The angle formed between these two lines is the Norberg angle.

the severity of the osteoarthritic changes. The most common surgical treatments are divided into those aiming to improve hip congruity (in an attempt to reduce the amount of future degenerative joint disease), and salvage procedures such as femoral head and neck excision and total hip replacement. The techniques that aim to improve hip congruity include pelvic osteotomies (triple and double pelvic osteotomies) and pubic symphysiodesis. Immature animals might benefit from pubic symphysiodesis. While this should ideally be performed at 12–16 weeks of age, it can be done in patients up to 22 weeks of age. Pelvic osteotomies are used in animals younger than 8–12 months of age, with mild to moderate hip laxity and minimal degenerative joint disease (minimal osteoarthritic changes). The techniques that aim to improve hip congruity therefore have a time window in which they can be beneficial for the patient. After that, other treatment options are more appropriate (either conservative treatment or salvage procedures). Only femoral head and neck excision will be discussed here, as the other techniques are beyond the scope of this book.

FEMORAL HEAD AND NECK EXCISION

INTRODUCTION

The femoral head and neck excision (FHNE) technique was first described in 1961 as a salvage procedure for patients with hip pathologies (Ormrod, 1961; Spreull, 1961).

> This procedure (also called femoral head and neck ostectomy or FHO) aims to eliminate the pain produced by bone-to-bone contact between the femoral head and the acetabulum during movement of the hip joint and weight-bearing.

Long-term stability of the limb relies on the development of a pseudoarthrosis with the joint capsule and periarticular fibrous tissue. The aim of this procedure is to provide a pain-free gait, and it is expected that patients will have some degree of gait abnormality after this procedure.

INDICATIONS

This technique is indicated in cases of nonreconstructable acetabular or femoral head or neck fractures. Animals with severe hip pain due to joint laxity or osteoarthritis which cannot be controlled with conservative treatment can also benefit from this procedure. Other indications include Legg–Calvé–Perthes disease, chronic hip luxation and recurrent acute hip luxation.

As some of the indications for this procedure are similar to those for a total hip replacement (THR), there is currently a debate as to whether the latter technique is more appropriate to treat the conditions previously mentioned. While a THR aims to return the patient to a normal gait and function, the aim of a FHNE is to provide a functional, pain-free gait, although gait abnormalities are expected. When deciding between these two surgical techniques, the clinical outcome should be weighed against the incidence and severity of possible surgical complications and the owner's financial constraints and expectations.

Another consideration when performing a FHNE is the patient's weight, as smaller patients (less than 15–17 kg in weight) have been reported to have a better outcome than heavier patients (Duff and Campbell, 1977), with a more variable outcome in animals over 20 kg (Anderson, 2011). A very good functional outcome of FHNE has been reported in cats (Yap et al., 2015). The idea that smaller patients perform better after a FHNE has, however, been challenged and it has been suggested that this technique should be limited to exceptional circumstances (Off and Matis, 1997).

Taking all these factors into consideration, the author currently recommends a THR in any patient over 15–20 kg, but will perform a FHNE in these patients when there are financial constraints or when the patient's owner does not want to risk the potential major complications associated with a THR. In smaller patients, the decision between a FHNE and a THR is more variable, and will depend on the owner's decision after discussing the desired functional outcome and the surgical risks of each technique.

SURGICAL PLANNING

Routine orthogonal pelvic radiographic views are usually taken to diagnose conditions in which a FHNE is a treatment option. These views are used to give a clear idea of the shape of the proximal femur, especially the shape of the greater trochanter and the location of the lesser trochanter, and to allow the surgeon to have a mental image of the location of the osteotomy in the patient's femur (Fig. 53).

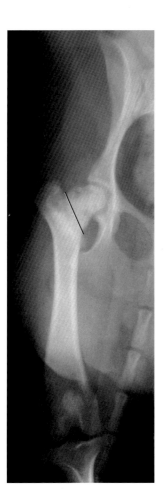

◀ Figure 53. Preoperative ventrodorsal radiograph of the pelvis of a dog diagnosed with Legg–Calvé–Perthes disease. The red line indicates the planned location of the osteotomy for a femoral head and neck excision.

SURGICAL TECHNIQUE

The approach to the hip joint is a standard craniolateral approach, although the skin incision does not need to be extended as far proximally and distally as in other procedures. In this technique, it is important to incise the medial insertion of the vastus lateralis muscle from the femoral neck to allow full exposure of the neck and better visualisation of the osteotomy site (Fig. 54). Once the femoral head is disarticulated, the limb is externally rotated and the femur is positioned so that both the femur and the patella are parallel to the floor and the patella is pointing towards the ceiling (Fig. 55).

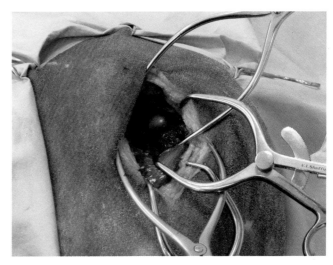

Figure 54. Exposure of the femoral head and neck for a femoral head and neck excision. The medial insertion of the vastus lateralis muscle has been incised and elevated for full exposure of the femoral neck.

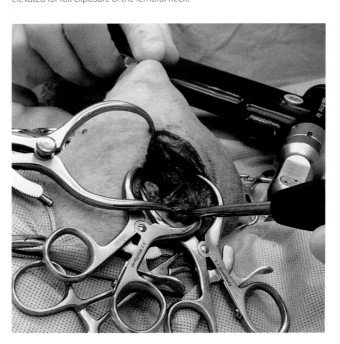

Figure 55. Once the round ligament has been transected, the limb is externally rotated until the femur and patella are parallel to the floor and the patella is pointing towards the ceiling. The surgeon's finger is pointing to the patella. ▶

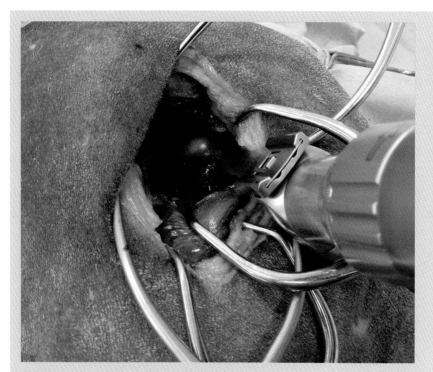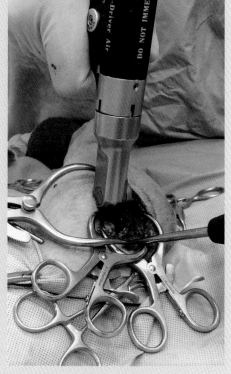

Figure 56. Two examples of incorrect positioning of the oscillating saw. The saw is slightly anteverted so that it is perpendicular to the femoral neck. This will inevitably leave a spur of the caudal neck.

A femoral head and neck ostectomy can be performed either with an oscillating power saw or with an osteotome and mallet. The author routinely uses an oscillating saw to have a more controlled osteotomy line and avoid bone spurs, irregular margins, and fissures that can develop when using an osteotome (O'Donnell et al., 2015). The ostectomy is performed as planned on the preoperative radiographs; it begins on the most lateral aspect of the intertrochanteric fossa (at the junction between the femoral neck and the greater trochanter) and is directed in a proximolateral to distomedial direction, ending just proximal to the lesser trochanter. It is extremely important not to leave any sharp ends at the osteotomy site as they will rub on the acetabular rim and interfere with the range of motion of the hip joint and with the formation of fibrous tissue between the acetabulum and the femur. Any sharp ends can be removed with a bone rasp or rongeurs. The natural tendency is to incorrectly antevert the osteotomy slightly, so that it is perpendicular to the femoral neck (Fig. 56). As the femoral neck has an anatomical anteversion, this will inevitably leave a spur of the caudal neck. The osteotomy must therefore be perpendicular to the floor, not to the femoral neck (Fig. 57).

Once the osteotomy is complete, the femoral head and neck are removed by grasping the head with pointed reduction forceps. Soft-tissue attachments are often present on the medial aspect of the femoral head and neck (joint capsule) and should be sharply dissected. Once the osteotomy site has been inspected to check for any bone spurs or femoral fissures (Fig. 58), the femoral external rotation is discontinued so that the femur moves back into its physiological position.

Interposition of tissue between the femur and the acetabulum (such as the deep gluteal, biceps femoris or rectus femoris muscles) has been described, but this is no longer standard practice. However, the author routinely performs a capsulorrhaphy if enough joint capsule is available. Manipulation of the hip through its full range of motion is performed to feel for any crepitus that would indicate an excessively long neck or the presence of bone spurs. If crepitus is present, the osteotomy should be performed more distally or any bone spurs should be removed with either a bone rasp or rongeurs. Closure of the surgical site is as previously described.

POSTOPERATIVE MANAGEMENT

Postoperative radiographs of the pelvis are indicated to assess the accuracy of the osteotomy and ensure there are no significant spurs at the osteotomy site (Fig. 59).

In order to achieve good hip range of motion, early controlled activity is recommended. Basic physiotherapy exercises (such as passive range of motion) should be performed

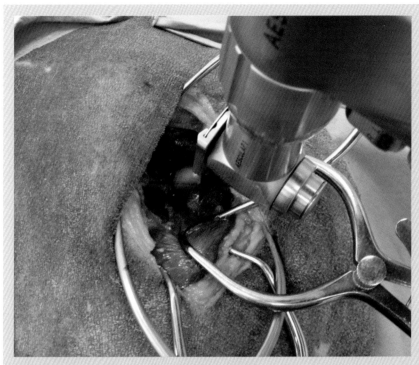

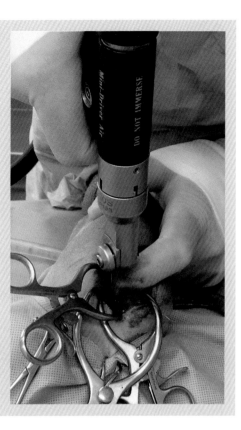

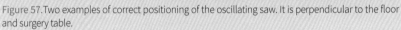

Figure 57. Two examples of correct positioning of the oscillating saw. It is perpendicular to the floor and surgery table.

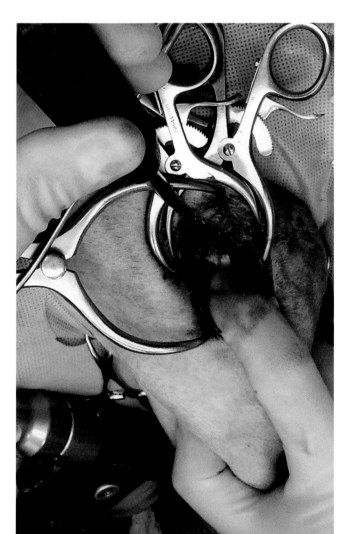

◀ Figure 58. Inspection of the femur for the presence of bone spurs or fissures once the ostectomy has been completed.

▼ Figure 59. Postoperative ventrodorsal radiograph of the pelvis after a femoral head and neck excision. This view is used to assess the accuracy of the osteotomy and ensure there are no significant spurs at the osteotomy site.

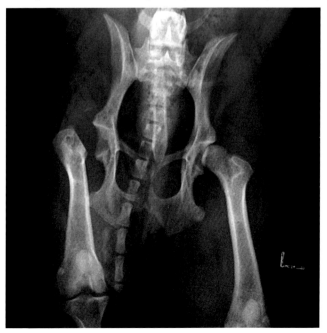

3–4 times a day, starting immediately after surgery. The patient can be kept on house rest and go for short lead walks (10–15 minutes) several times per day. Any vigorous exercise should be avoided. Hydrotherapy can be very beneficial once the skin sutures have been removed 10–12 days after surgery, at which point exercise can be increased to as much as the patient is comfortable with. Physiotherapy exercises should be continued until the patient is fully weight-bearing and using the limb consistently.

OUTCOME

Assessing the outcome of this procedure is difficult as all patients are expected to have some degree of gait abnormality due to limb shortening, reduced range of motion and muscle atrophy. This is considered a mechanical lameness and the patient should be pain free. Therefore, using subjective gait analysis to assess the outcome of this surgery might be misleading, and assessing the functional outcome is probably more relevant in these patients.

As previously mentioned, several factors might influence the outcome in these patients. Patients with greater body weight, animals older than 1 year, and those with a significant degree of muscle wasting prior to surgery have a potentially worse outcome (Rawson et al., 2005; Anderson, 2011; Wong, 2016). The final degree of improvement may only be achieved after 6–8 months, but younger patients improve faster (Berzon et al., 1980; Penwick, 1992; DeCamp et al., 2016).

The overall outcome of this procedure is very variable, with good to excellent results reported in 63–83 % of cases. Although in one study, 96 % of the owners were satisfied with the procedure, 56 % of the patients had persistent lameness and 32 % had persistent pain (Off, 1997). In this study, the functional outcome combining all sizes of dogs was good in 38 %, satisfactory in 20 % and poor in 42 % of the cases, with the owners reporting that their dogs avoided trotting (Off and Matis, 1997). Another study using FHNE for treatment of Legg–Calvé–Perthes disease reported that 66 % of the patients had a good to excellent outcome, although some patients had mild intermittent lameness episodes (Piek et al., 1996).

It seems that the functional outcome of FHNE is more predictable in cats than in dogs. In the study by Off and Matis (1997), 73 % of the cats had a reduced range of motion of the hip, 27 % exhibited pain on passive range of motion, and 47 % had muscle atrophy. However, none of the 15 cats examined had clinical lameness at long-term follow-up and the outcome was considered satisfactory. A recent study has also demonstrated good to excellent long-term outcomes in 18 cats after FHNE, with almost all cats going back to performing their normal daily activities after a 1- to 2-month recovery period (Yap et al., 2015). The main change noticed in this study was a reduction in the height of the jump in 39 % of the cats. However, other reports have suggested that the outcome in cats is also unpredictable and that THR has an overall better functional outcome than FHNE in this species (Liska et al., 2009).

COMPLICATIONS

Surgical complications are uncommon following FHNE; the most common is persistent lameness due to bone spurs at the osteotomy site producing bone-to-bone contact.

Other reported complications include continuing lameness, discomfort after exercise, muscle atrophy, stiffness, difficulty jumping, limb shortening, patellar luxation, and decreased range of motion of the hip joint.

Other less common complications include sciatic nerve entrapment, injury to the sciatic nerve during or after surgery, and fractures of the greater trochanter or femoral shaft during the ostectomy (Berzon et al., 1980; Jeffery, 1993; Wong, 2016).

LEGG–CALVÉ–PERTHES DISEASE

Legg–Calvé–Perthes disease is an aseptic avascular necrosis of the femoral head of unknown origin. It is more common in young, small-breed dogs (especially Terriers), and progresses in three phases: an initial phase of necrosis of the femoral head trabeculae, followed by a phase of femoral subchondral bone collapse and fragmentation, and a final phase of reossification due to a revascularisation process of the femoral head (Towle, 2012). The resulting femoral changes cause joint incongruity and degenerative joint disease in the hip.

Clinical signs include episodes of acute or chronic lameness with pain and crepitus when manipulating the affected hip and moving it through its range of motion. Patients are usually very young (less than 1 year of age) and those with chronic lameness will present with muscle atrophy of the affected limb. There is no sex predisposition, and the condition can be bilateral in up to 16.5 % of cases (Lee, 1969).

Radiographs of the pelvis are commonly diagnostic of this condition (Figs. 60 and 61), and computed tomography can be a useful diagnostic tool in the early stages of the disease. The radiographic appearance of the femoral head depends on the phase of the disease. The femoral head may have a mottled appearance due to focal bone lysis in the early stages of the disease, or be collapsed and deformed with thickening of the femoral neck in more advanced cases. In some instances, a femoral head or femoral neck fracture may be found.

Treatment of this condition involves salvage procedures such as a FHNE (see *Femoral head and neck excision*, p. 22) or THR. Histopathological analysis of the femoral head is recommended to confirm the presumptive clinical diagnosis.

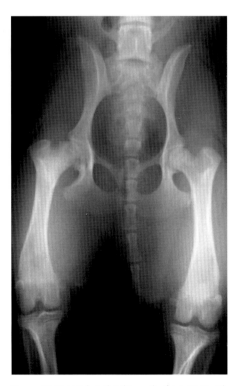

Figure 60. Ventrodorsal radiograph of a patient with right Legg–Calvé–Perthes disease. Note the mottled appearance of the femoral head, which corresponds to the phase of trabecular necrosis of the femoral head.

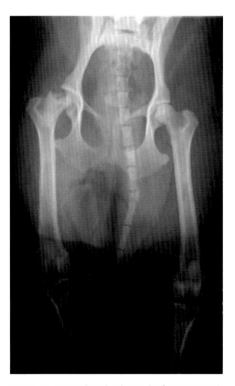

Figure 61. Ventrodorsal radiograph of a patient with right Legg–Calvé–Perthes disease. Severe lytic changes with an abnormal contour of the femoral head are observed in this patient.

02
THE STIFLE

PATELLAR LUXATION

INTRODUCTION

The extensor mechanism of the stifle is composed of the quadriceps muscle group (vastus medialis, lateralis, intermedius and rectus femoris), the patella, the patellar tendon, and the patellar retinaculum and its insertion at the tibial tuberosity (Fig. 1). It allows stifle extension and therefore forms part of the weight-bearing mechanism of the pelvic limb in the standing animal, and it facilitates propulsion during ambulation.

Patellar luxation is one of the most common orthopaedic conditions in the dog (Johnson et al., 1994; Ness et al., 1996). It is a developmental condition with an inherited component; anatomical deformities that lead to an abnormal extensor mechanism tend to be present at birth and these progress as the dog grows. Traumatic patellar luxation has been reported but has a significantly lower incidence. Patellar luxation can be classified as medial (MPL), lateral (LPL), and bidirectional.

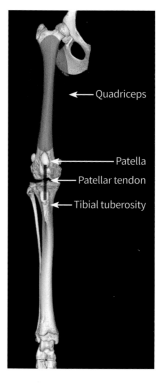

Figure 1. Quadriceps/extensor mechanism.

Different grades of luxation have been described by several authors (Roush, 1993):

- Grade 1: The patella can be manually luxated but returns to its normal position when released.
- Grade 2: The patella luxates upon stifle flexion or manual manipulation and remains luxated until the stifle is extended or the patella is replaced manually.
- Grade 3: The patella luxates continually. It can be replaced but reluxates spontaneously when manual pressure is removed.
- Grade 4: The patella is permanently luxated and cannot be replaced.

Anatomical abnormalities in the extensor mechanism are more pronounced in higher-grade luxations (Fig. 2). Several factors have been reported to increase the likelihood of patellar luxation, including coxa vara and reduced anteversion (relative retroversion) of the femoral neck (Putnam, 1968). Dogs with radiographic signs of patella alta (ratio of patellar tendon length (L) to patellar length (P) >2) were more likely to suffer from MPL (Mostafa et al., 2008) (Fig. 3).

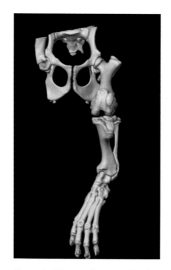

Figure 2. CT scan of a young Dachshund with bone deformities, lateral patellar luxation and pes varus.

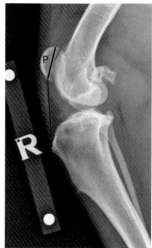

Figure 3. Mediolateral radiograph of a stifle showing the ratio of patellar tendon length (L) to patellar length (P).

Moreover, radiographic evaluation in a study by Soparat et al. (2012) in Pomeranian dogs with MPL revealed that the incidence of femoral varus was significantly higher in high-grade luxations (3–4) than in lower-grade luxations (1–2).

The incidence of concurrent patellar luxation and cranial cruciate ligament disease has been reported in one study as 25 % (Campbell et al., 2010). Older patients and patients with a higher degree of luxation had a higher incidence of cranial cruciate ligament disease. Other papers have reported that middle-aged dogs both with and without MPL had a similar prevalence of cranial cruciate ligament disease, throwing into doubt whether there is a causal relationship between the two conditions (Hayes et al., 2013).

INDICATIONS FOR SURGERY

Surgical management of MPL is recommended for older patients with clinical signs of lameness or chronic pain associated with luxation. The most common presentation is that of a young to older animal with grade 2–3 patellar luxation. Older patients with a chronic low-grade MPL and acute clinical deterioration should be thoroughly evaluated for the presence of concurrent cranial cruciate ligament disease.

Very immature patients with pronounced anatomical abnormalities of the extensor mechanism would benefit from early surgical intervention. These patients may require a second or more surgical procedures when osseous maturity is reached.

Traumatic patellar luxation is an uncommon cause of patellar luxation in dogs and is seen occasionally in cats. Surgical intervention is warranted and generally involves medial/lateral retinaculum reconstruction.

SURGICAL PLANNING

The radiographic examination should include orthogonal views of the femur and tibia.

> It is essential to properly evaluate the position of the patella and tibial tuberosity, as well as the degree of degenerative joint disease and skeletal deformities.

Excluding other concurrent conditions is also paramount. In patients with concurrent cranial cruciate ligament disease, mediolateral radiographs tend to show more pronounced signs suggestive of stifle effusion (cranial displacement of the infrapatellar fat pad and caudal displacement of the

subgastrocnemius fascia), as well as osteophytes cranial to the tibial plateau at the level of insertion of the cranial cruciate ligament (see Fig. 4 in *Cranial cruciate ligament disease - Clinical history, physical examination and diagnosis*, p. 43).

It is the author's preference to obtain craniocaudal radiographs from hip to hock (Fig. 4) and mediolateral radiographs of the femur.

> Radiographic positioning can greatly affect the apparent degree of femoral deformities.

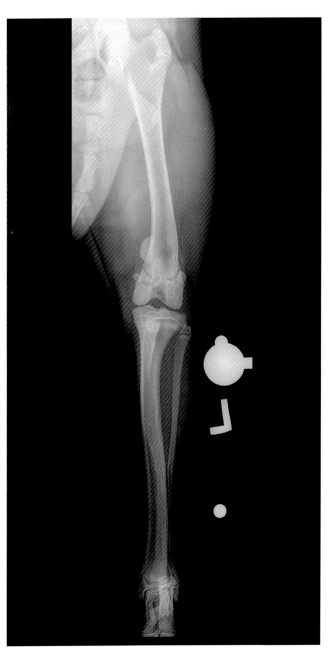

Figure 4. Craniocaudal view from the coxofemoral to the talocrural joint. Ideal for first approximation to limb alignment.

The presence of the "double condyle sign" on medio-lateral radiographs of the femur suggests there is femoral deformity (Fig. 5). One femoral condyle projected distal to the other may be suggestive of femoral varus/valgus, while one femoral condyle appearing cranial to the other may be suggestive of torsional deformity. When in doubt, remember that the long digital extensor fossa is found on the lateral aspect of the lateral femoral condyle; this will facilitate identification of the latter on mediolateral radiographs of the distal femur. Evaluation of the femoral varus angle using CT has been validated and is the author's preference to assess and plan the surgery of femoral deformities (Oxley, 2013a). It is strongly recommended in high-grade patellar luxation. Normal femoral angles have been compiled for some breeds of dogs by Petazzoni et al. (2008) and can be used as a reference.

Management of femoral deformities with corrective osteo-tomies is beyond the scope of this book. Individual evaluation of the position of the tibial tuberosity, depth of the femoral trochlea, torsional and frontal planes deformities are essential to determine the specific surgical procedure required for each case of patellar luxation. A singular cut-off value for distal femoral varus necessitating distal femoral ostectomy cannot be advocated. Large-breed dogs seem to have poorer outcomes with wide distal femoral varus angle without femoral corrections.

Management of patients with bilateral patellar luxation can be performed by staged or simultaneous surgical procedures. No significant differences were reported in terms of overall complication rate between simultaneous bilateral repair of MPL and unilateral or staged bilateral surgery in dogs weighing less than 15 kg (Gallegos, 2016). It is the author's preference to perform staged procedures unless there are financial or animal welfare constraints.

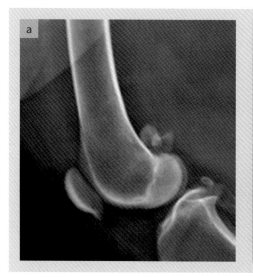 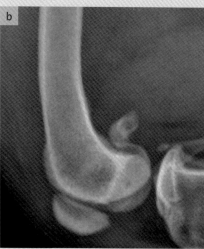

Figure 5. Mediolateral view of the distal femur in a dog with perfectly superimposed lateral and medial aspects of the femoral condyle (a). "Double condyle" sign suggestive of distal femoral deformity (b).

SURGICAL TECHNIQUE

The author positions the dog in dorsal recumbency. Following surgical preparation of the limb, standard four-quarter draping is performed and an adhesive iodine-impregnated drape is applied (Fig. 6).

Using a lateral parapatellar approach, a parapatellar arthrotomy is performed.

> Assessment of the cranial cruciate ligament is indicated in all cases. Flexion of the stifle and retraction of the infrapatellar fat pad facilitates cranial cruciate ligament examination.

Concurrent management of MPL and cranial cruciate ligament disease has been reported with several techniques which are beyond the scope of this book.

The depth of the femoral trochlea and state of the cartilage are assessed (Fig. 7). Dogs with a high-grade luxation and extensive cartilage erosion may require patellar groove replacement.

TROCHLEAR GROOVE DEEPENING PROCEDURES

The author prefers to perform trochlear block recession (Fig. 8) rather than wedge recession (Fig. 9), as it achieves a higher proximal patellar depth with greater resistance to patellar luxation in an extended position (Johnson et al., 2001). For small patients, a wedge recession trochleoplasty (sulcoplasty) subjectively offers a lower risk of iatrogenic trochlear fractures. The depth of the trochlea after surgery should cover 33 % of the patella in a craniocaudal plane.

For both trochlear block recession and wedge recession, a thin power blade (microsagittal saw blade, Fig. 10) or surgical saw are used (Fig. 11).

The author prefers to outline the block/wedge initially with a number 11 scalpel blade.

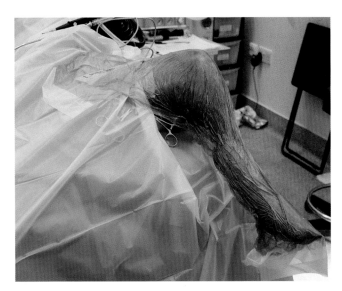

Figure 6. Patient in dorsal recumbency after draping and application of an iodine-impregnated incision drape.

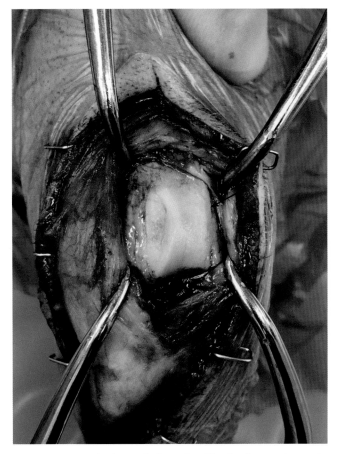

Figure 7. Intraoperative image of a femoral trochlea. Cartilage erosion can be seen on the proximomedial aspect of the trochlea (black arrow).

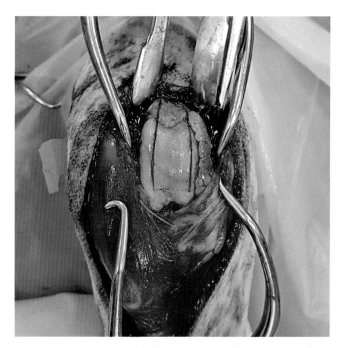

Figure 8. Intraoperative image of a block recession trochleoplasty after performing the abaxial cuts.

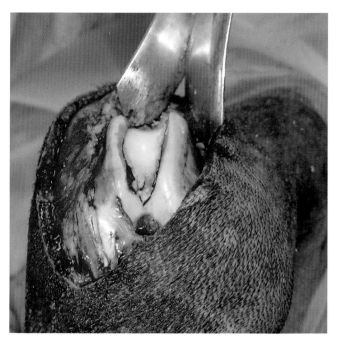

Figure 9. Intraoperative image of a distal femur after performing a wedge recession and placing the autograft.

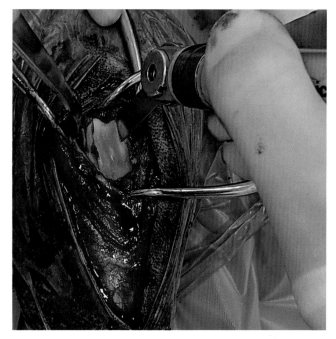

Figure 10. Example of the use of a power blade to perform a block recession trochleoplasty.

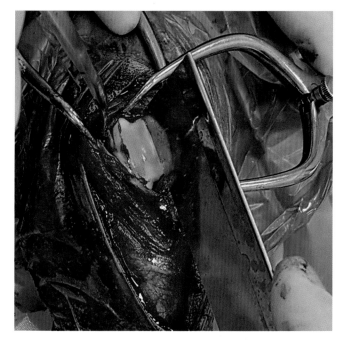

Figure 11. Example of the use of a surgical saw to cut the abaxial extent of the graft for a block recession trochleoplasty.

Block recession trochleoplasty

In a block recession trochleoplasty, the distal end of the trochlear block including the sulcus reaches just above the intercondylar femoral notch. Care must be taken in the most proximal portion of the trochlea as luxation is generally seen in this region when the stifle is extended. The author prefers to extend the trochlear surgery 2–3 mm proximal to the location of the patella with the stifle in extension to minimise the likelihood of reluxation. The abaxial cuts are angled approximately 10 degrees from the axial plane, ensuring that the width of the block is greater than that of the patella. The base of the autograft is then removed using a high-speed drill or rongeurs. For additional depth, the cancellous bed is deepened with the use of a modular osteotome (Fig. 12) and/or high-speed drill (Fig. 13).

Digital pressure is applied to fit the autograft in the recipient bed (Fig. 14). In large dogs, gentle hammering of the autograft, using a swab to protect the cartilage, can be performed to improve its sitting. Rotating the autograft 180 degrees before reducing it into the graft bed may give additional trochlear depth and a better fit. If the autograft is deemed excessively mobile, a small Kirshner wire can be used, passing from the lateral aspect of the distal femur, crossing the autograft, and exiting on the medial aspect of the distal femur to fix the autograft in position and minimise dislodgement.

Wedge recession trochleoplasty

In this technique, a V-shaped wedge that includes the sulcus is removed from the trochlea. Additional widening of the defect by cutting out a portion of the remaining trochlea parallel to one of the sides of V-shaped wedge is performed (Figs. 15 and 16).

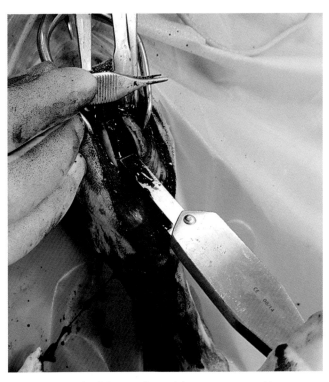

Figure 12. Example of the use of a modular osteotome to achieve an even deeper trochlear groove after a trochlear block recession.

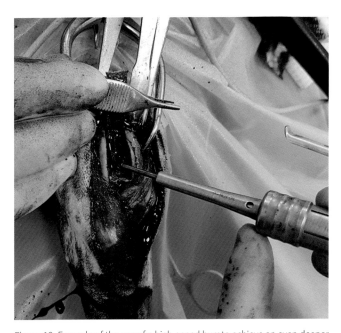

Figure 13. Example of the use of a high-speed burr to achieve an even deeper trochlear groove after a trochlear block recession.

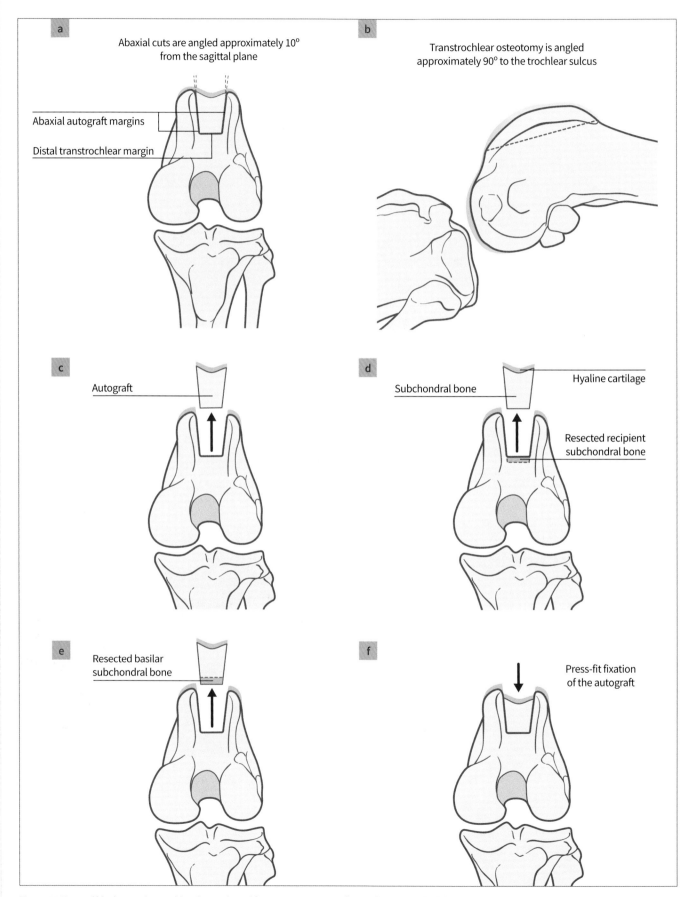

a — Abaxial cuts are angled approximately 10° from the sagittal plane

Abaxial autograft margins

Distal transtrochlear margin

b — Transtrochlear osteotomy is angled approximately 90° to the trochlear sulcus

c — Autograft

d — Subchondral bone

Hyaline cartilage

Resected recipient subchondral bone

e — Resected basilar subchondral bone

f — Press-fit fixation of the autograft

Figure 14. Femoral block recession trochleoplasty. Adapted from: Fossum TW, *Small Animal Surgery*, 3rd ed. (2007).

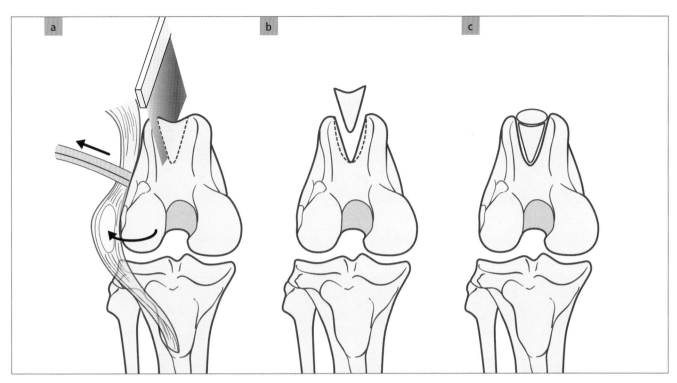

Figure 15. Wedge recession sulcoplasty technique. Resection of the V-shaped wedge (a), additional widening of the defect to facilitate deeper sitting of the autograft (b), and autograft (wedge) back in position showing adequate depth of the groove for the patella to sit in (c). Adapted from: Fossum TW, *Small Animal Surgery*, 3rd ed. (2007).

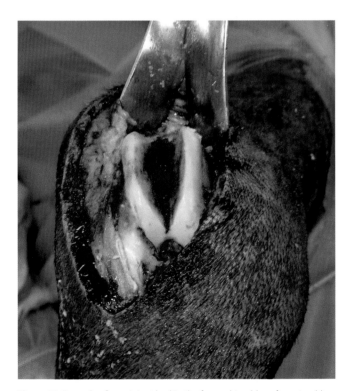

Figure 16. Example of a recipient bed in the femoral trochlea after a trochlear wedge recession.

TROCHLEAR CHONDROPLASTY

Trochlear chondroplasty is performed in immature dogs (<10 months of age) whose trochlear cartilage is thick enough to be elevated without breaking. A number 11 scalpel blade is used to outline and elevate a cartilage flap of similar proportions to the block recession. Once the cartilage flap is elevated, the groove in the subchondral cancellous bone is deepened with a high-speed drill or rongeurs. Once the depth is adequate, the cartilage flap is press-fitted back into the recipient bed.

TIBIAL TUBEROSITY TRANSPOSITION

Tibial tuberosity transposition (TTT) is performed in all those cases in which the tibial tuberosity is not aligned with the patella. The direction of the patellar tendon running from the cranial pole of the patella to the tibial tuberosity is used to evaluate alignment.

A medial approach to the tibial tuberosity is used by extending the lateral parapatellar approach cranially to the proximal aspect of the tibia; folding the skin should provide enough exposure to perform a tibial tuberosity osteotomy.

Planning the size of the tibial tuberosity osteotomy is recommended to avoid trauma to the cranial cruciate ligament, long digital extensor tendon, or patellar tendon (Fig. 17).

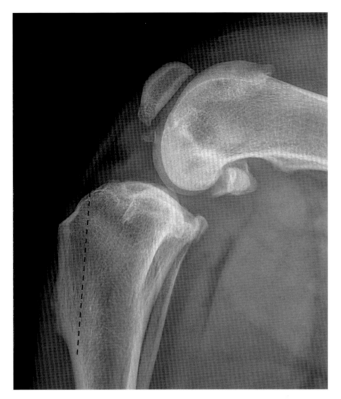

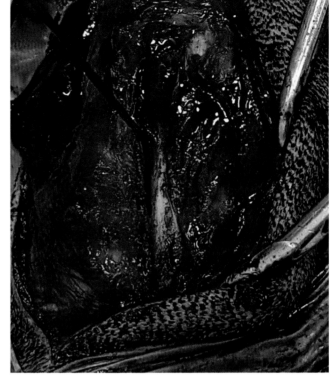

Figure 17. Example of a tibial tuberosity osteotomy for transposition (dotted red line). It is important to avoid damaging the long digital extensor tendon, the patellar tendon and the cranial cruciate ligament with the osteotomy.

Figure 18. Use of a Kirschner wire to immobilise the tibial tuberosity laterally after temporary transposition.

Generally, the width of the tibial tuberosity osteotomy at the level of the insertion of the patellar tendon should not exceed 33 % of the craniocaudal width of the tibia at this level.

Following the landmarks obtained from preoperative radiographs, monopolar cautery and a calliper are used to outline the portion of the tibial tuberosity to be excised with a microsagittal blade.

> The author usually prefers to perform an incomplete osteotomy at the distal aspect as this may provide a tension-band effect. Extension of the stifle should facilitate transposition of the tuberosity after the osteotomy.

Once adequate translation has been achieved, a temporary Kirschner wire can be positioned in the recipient bed to act as a stopper so the alignment of the extensor mechanism can be assessed more easily before final stabilisation (Fig. 18).

Once good alignment is confirmed, a definitive Kirschner wire is driven proximal to the insertion of the patellar tendon (Fig. 19) in a cranioproximal to caudodistal direction. The size of the Kirschner wire should be less than one-third of the width of the tibial tuberosity at this point. For pin orientation, remember that the bone stock (bone that provides the interface for implant fixation) on the tibia would be medial to the laterally translated portion of the tuberosity. A second Kirschner wire is driven parallel to the first one in large dogs or distal to it in small-breed dogs (Fig. 20). Cerclage wire of a similar size to the most proximal Kirschner wire is chosen to create a tension-band construct (Fig. 21).

Distalisation of the tibial tuberosity has been reported for management of patella alta (Segal, 2012).

Soft tissue techniques

Imbrication of the lateral retinaculum for MPL and medial retinaculum for LPL is generally performed. Horizontal Cushing's or modified Mayo sutures are placed in an interrupted pattern (Figs. 22 and 23). Preplacing of the sutures facilitates closure. The degree of imbrication is subjectively assessed, and sutures modified depending on the tracking of the patella after suture placement.

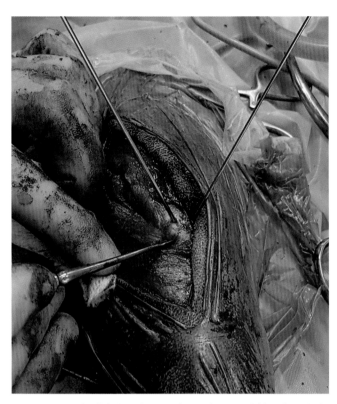

Figure 19. Example of ideal localisation of a Kirschner wire (of less than 1/3 the size of the width of the tibial tuberosity) proximal to the insertion of the patellar tendon to secure it after transposition.

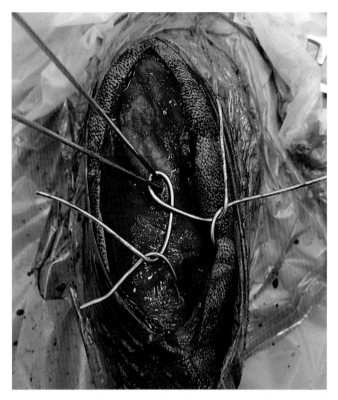

Figure 20. Example of use of a second Kirschner wire to secure the transposed tibial tuberosity. Due to the small size of the patient, the second Kirschner wire is placed distal to the first one.

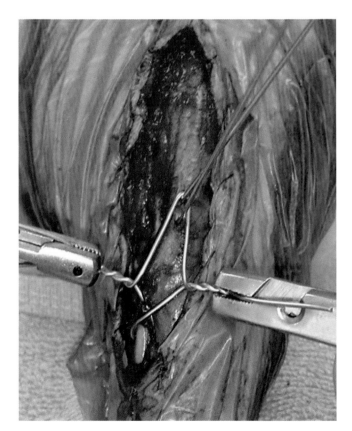

Figure 21. Example of the use of Kirschner wires and cerclage to create a tension-band construct.

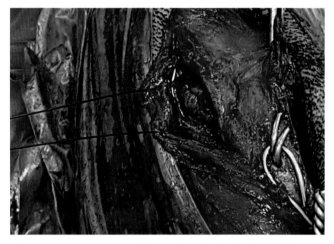

Figure 22. Intraoperative image of lateral retinaculum imbrication with the use of a Cushing's suture pattern.

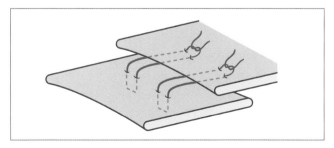

Figure 23. Modified Mayo mattress suture.

In high-grade MPL with substantial soft tissue adaptations and internal rotation of the stifle, release of the pes anserinus on the medial aspect of the proximal tibia and a releasing incision between the vastus medialis and rectus femoris may need to be performed.

Closure of the tissues on the medial aspect can be performed with loose sutures to avoid dead space and lateral patella luxation. External rotation of the stifle using a lateral fabellotibial suture (see *Extracapsular repair*, p. 44) could be combined with soft tissue release in cases with excessive internal stifle rotation during maximal stifle flexion. Patellar tracking is evaluated. Closure is performed as per routine in three layers. Postoperative radiographs are taken to assess the apparatus and positioning of the patella.

POSTOPERATIVE MANAGEMENT

Perioperative antibiotic therapy is given to all patients and discontinued after the surgical procedure is complete. A short course of oral nonsteroidal anti-inflammatory drugs (NSAIDs) is provided for 14 days. The limb is not usually bandaged and it is recommended that cryotherapy is applied every 4–6 h for the first 72 hours after surgery.

Strict rest is prescribed for 6 weeks (confinement in a big cage or small room). No jumping, running, walking on slippery surfaces, steps or stairs or off-lead exercise are allowed. The patient can go outside on the lead for 10 minutes 3–4 times a day for toilet purposes. The skin sutures or staples are removed after 12 days. Follow-up radiographs are taken after 6 weeks under heavy sedation (Fig. 24).

Provided there is evidence of advanced healing and no implant-related issues, lead exercise can be increased by 5 minutes per walk on a weekly basis over a 4-week period, followed by slow reintroduction of off-lead exercise over an additional 4-week period. Physiotherapy can be considered after the 6-week follow-up visit.

OUTCOME

The outcome correlates with the grade of luxation (Remedios et al., 1992), with lower grades having higher chances of excellent long-term outcome. Hans et al. (2016) reported full function in 42.6 % of dogs (n=47 total stifles) after surgical management of grade 4 MPL, while 4.5 % had an acceptable outcome and 17 % had an unacceptable outcome.

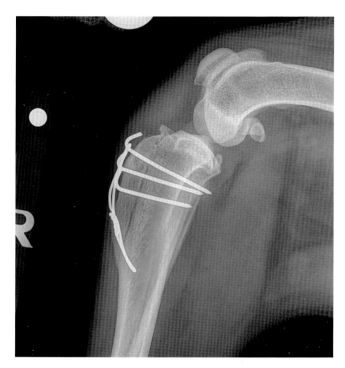

Figure 24. Six-week postoperative mediolateral radiograph of a stifle after MPL surgery (tibial tuberosity transposition, block recession trochleoplasty and lateral imbrication). In this case, an additional Kirschner wire was driven due to the large size of the patient. Signs of progressive bone union are seen at the osteotomy site and at the femoral trochlea.

COMPLICATIONS

An overall complication rate of 18–25 % has been reported (Gallegos, 2016; Hans et al., 2016; Kalff et al., 2014).

Major complications were recently reviewed (Cashmore et al., 2014) and reported in 18.5 % of the dogs that had undergone surgery for management of MPL. Implant-related complications, patellar reluxation and tibial tuberosity avulsion were the most commonly encountered.

Major complications were associated with corrective osteotomies (Hans et al., 2016).

According to recent literature (Cashmore et al., 2014), a combination of trochleoplasty and tibial tuberosity transposition reduces the likelihood of patellar reluxation by 5.1 times.

Tibial tuberosity avulsion was 11.1 times more likely to occur when using one Kirschner wire instead of two and none of the cases in which a tension-band construct was used showed avulsion of the tibial tuberosity.

> The author prefers to use a tension-band construct with two Kirschner wires and to perform trochlear surgery in almost all cases.

CRANIAL CRUCIATE LIGAMENT DISEASE

INTRODUCTION

CRANIAL CRUCIATE LIGAMENT: ANATOMY AND FUNCTION

The cruciate ligaments are located centrally in the intercondylar fossa. They limit cranial and caudal translation of the tibia on the femur. The cranial cruciate ligament runs from the caudomedial part of the lateral condyle of the femur diagonally across the intercondylar fossa to the cranial intercondylar area of the tibia (Gordon-Evans et al., 2013). The cranial cruciate ligament is composed of two bands: the craniomedial and the caudolateral (Fig. 1). The craniomedial band is taut in flexion and extension, whereas the caudolateral band is only taut in extension. This has clinical relevance in cases with partial cruciate ligament rupture during physical examination. In addition to limiting tibial translation on the femur, the cranial cruciate ligament also limits internal rotation of the tibia relative to the femur.

The caudal cruciate ligament runs from the lateral surface of the medial condyle caudodistally to the lateral edge of the popliteal notch of the tibia. Both cranial and caudal cruciate ligaments are intra-articular, but extrasynovial, structures.

Cranial cruciate ligament (CrCL) disease is multifactorial, with several factors having been reported to influence its incidence, including genetics, conformation factors (genu varum, internal femoral rotation, medial patellar luxation, proximal tibial deformities, intercondylar notch stenosis and excessive tibial plateau angle), early neutering, excessive bodyweight and sedentary lifestyle, dynamic muscle imbalance and an inflammatory component. Together, these lead to a disparity between the mechanical forces placed on the ligament and its ability to sustain loads, with eventual ligament rupture and development of degenerative joint disease (Griffon, 2010). Cranial cruciate ligament disease is the most common orthopaedic condition of the dog stifle (Innes et al., 2000; Aragon and Budsberg, 2005). It is commonly seen in older dogs, with most cases having a degenerative aetiology although traumatic cases are sometimes seen. Hyperextension or excessive internal rotation with the stifle flexed are the movements most likely to cause tearing of the CrCL (Gordon-Evans, 2013).

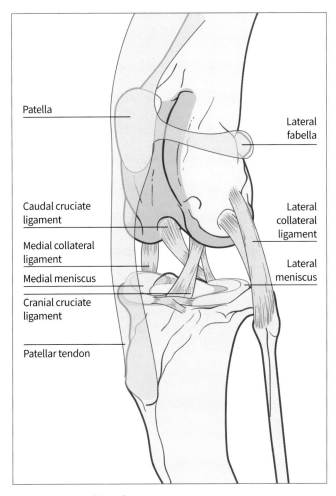

Figure 1. Anatomy of the stifle joint.

The incidence of CrCL disease has doubled over the last 30 years (Witsberger et al., 2008). The economic implications of managing CrCL disease in dog are substantial and were estimated in 2003 to be 1.3 billion dollars annually in the United States (Wilke et al., 2005).

CLINICAL HISTORY, PHYSICAL EXAMINATION AND DIAGNOSIS

Dogs with CrCL disease generally present with hindlimb lameness of different degrees. When acute full rupture of the CrCL happens, dogs are more likely to manifest a high-grade pelvic limb lameness or even non-weight-bearing lameness. The degree of lameness tends to improve over time.

Despite improvement, full resolution is not generally seen in dogs heavier than 15 kg (Vasseur, 1984).

For patients with partial CrCL disease, clinical presentation varies from mild to moderate weight-bearing lameness that worsens after strenuous exercise and with stiffness commonly seen after rest. Other common differential diagnoses to consider in the patient with pelvic limb lameness are patellar luxation, degenerative lumbosacral stenosis, hip dysplasia/coxofemoral arthritis, stifle osteochondrosis/chondritis dissecans, common calcaneal tendinopathy, caudal cruciate ligament disease, lateralised intervertebral disc disease in the lumbar spine, long digital extensor pathology (large and giant breed dogs), neoplasia, fibrotic myopathies and other arthropathies.

Administration of NSAIDs and rest generally improve the severity of lameness and general function in the dog with CrCL disease but resolution is often not seen. Meniscal injuries and complete rupture of the CrCL can lead to acute deterioration.

During physical examination, pain is generally seen on stifle flexion and extension. Muscle mass atrophy is commonly seen on the affected limb (quadriceps and hamstring muscles) and can vary from mild to severe depending on chronicity. Patients with stifle effusion tend to have an illdefined margin of the patellar tendon during stifle palpation. Palpable fibrosis on the medial aspect of the stifle is generally found in chronic cases (medial buttress). A definitive diagnosis is commonly made during physical examination in patients with unstable cruciate disease by the cranial drawer and/or tibial compression tests (Figs. 2 and 3). It is paramount to perform the cranial drawer test with the stifle in flexion, in a neutral position and in extension. Patients with partial rupture of the CrCL involving the craniomedial band would only have a positive cranial drawer sign with a flexed stifle, whereas a positive cranial drawer sign with an extended stifle would suggest rupture of the craniomedial and caudolateral bands. Dogs with chronic disease may have a negative tibial compression test/cranial drawer.

The radiographic workup for patient with suspected stifle disease should include a ventrodorsal view of the pelvis with the hips in extension, a lateral view of the pelvis, and orthogonal radiographs of the affected and contralateral stifles. Radiographic signs suggestive of CrCL disease are tibial subluxation on mediolateral radiographs, the presence of a stifle opacity displacing the infrapatellar fat pad cranially and subgastrocnemius fascia caudally, and the presence of periarticular osteophytes and enthesophytes at the level of insertion of the CrCL cranial to the tibial plateau (Fig. 4).

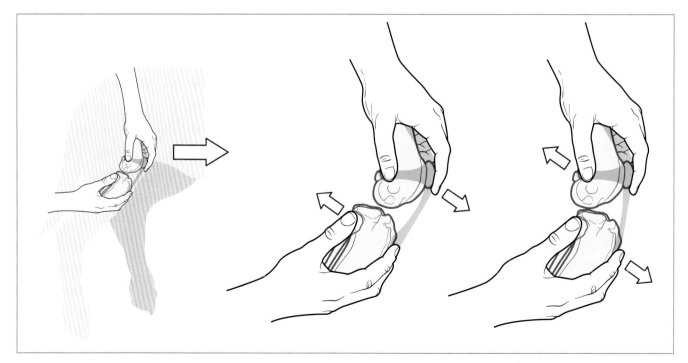

Figure 2. Cranial drawer test. The index and thumb of one hand are placed on the cranial and caudal aspects of the distal femur respectively. The other hand is positioned with the index finger on the cranial aspect of the tibial tuberosity and the thumb on the caudal aspect of the tibia. With the stifle in flexion, cranial force is applied on the tibia with the hand. The same manoeuvre is repeated with the stifle in extension. A cranial displacement of the tibia with respect to the femur is considered a positive test.

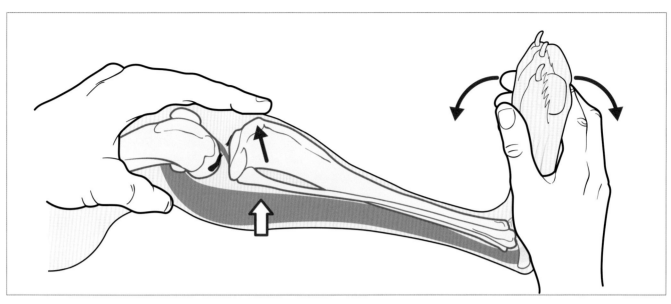

Figure 3. Tibial compression test. The index of one hand is placed on the cranial aspect of the tibial tuberosity with the thumb of the same hand on the back of the stifle. The second hand flexes the hock with proximal compression of the tibia. A positive compression test would elicit cranial translation of the tibia, and therefore cranial movement of the index finger placed on the tibial tuberosity.

Dogs with stable CrCL disease (negative cranial drawer sign and tibial compression tests) are more challenging to diagnose. Definitive diagnosis can be confirmed by MRI and/or by surgical exploration (arthroscopy/arthrotomy). Despite the reported sensitivity of high power field MRI for detection of CrCL disease (Barrett et al., 2009), its limited availability and associated costs precludes a more widespread use of this technique (Figs. 5, 6 and 7). When dogs present with the typical history, physical and radiographic signs of CrCL disease as described here, it is the author's general recommendation to perform stifle arthroscopy/arthrotomy to obtain a definitive diagnosis and to proceed with surgical management when appropriate. Stifle arthrocentesis is advised for all patients with stifle pain on manipulation, negative tibial compression/cranial drawer tests and radiographic signs suggestive of stifle effusion.

Dogs with bilateral CrCL disease can present with severe difficulties in ambulation and may be confused with patients with neurological disease. Full neurological examination with particular attention paid to postural reactions and spinal reflexes is strongly recommended to distinguish between orthopaedic and neurological disease.

Contralateral CrCL disease after confirmation of CrCL disease is very common. In Labrador Retrievers, Buote et al. (2009) reported that contralateral CrCL deficiency would be predicted to occur within 5.5 months of first diagnosis in 50% of cases.

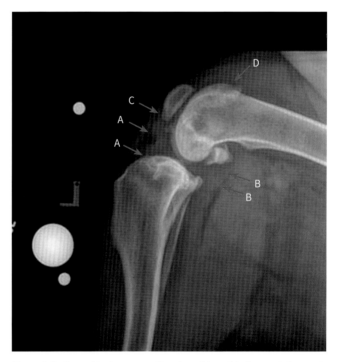

Figure 4. Radiographic signs suggestive of cranial cruciate ligament disease. A, presence of enthesophytes cranial to the tibial plateau at the level of insertion of the cranial cruciate ligament; B, increased opacity suggestive of stifle effusion on mediolateral radiographs (cranial displacement of infrapatellar fat pad and caudal displacement of subgastrocnemius fascia); C, osteophytes at the apex of the patella; D, osteophytes on the femoral trochlea.

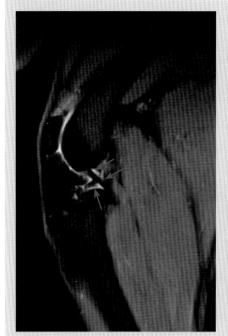

Figure 5. Sagittal view of a proton density MRI sequence of a nonpathological stifle. Note the homogeneous hypointense texture of the cranial and caudal cruciate ligaments (arrows).

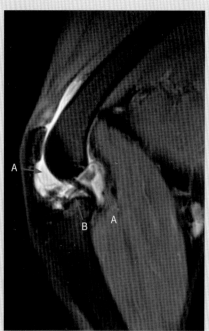

Figure 6. Sagittal view of a proton density MRI sequence of a dog with cranial cruciate ligament disease. Note the presence of hyperintense (white) signal suggestive of joint effusion (A) and a non-homogeneous cranial cruciate ligament (B) with hyperintense signal suggestive of cranial cruciate ligament disease.

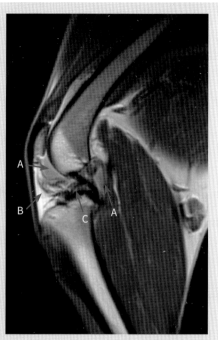

Figure 7. Sagittal view of a T2-weighed MRI sequence of a dog with cranial cruciate ligament disease. Note the presence of hyperintense (white) signal suggestive of joint effusion (A) that is relatively hypointense to the infrapatellar fat pad (B), and a nonhomogeneous cranial cruciate ligament (C) with hyperintense signal suggestive of cranial cruciate ligament disease.

SURGICAL AND NONSURGICAL MANAGEMENT

Nonsurgical management of dogs with CrCL disease has been investigated and is most commonly recommended for dogs weighing less than 15 to 20 kg, (Vasseur, 1984; Comerford et al., 2013) although an improvement in lameness with nonsurgical management of CrCL disease has been reported for dogs weighing more than 20 kg (Chauvet et al., 1996; Wucherer et al., 2013). More recently, Hart et al. (2016) compared owner satisfaction between tibial plateau levelling osteotomy (TPLO) and a custom-made stifle orthosis for management of medium and large-breed dogs with CrCL disease. More than 85 % of respondents in both groups would choose the selected treatment again. Eleven percent of the dogs that initially had an orthosis required surgery, while 46 % of dogs treated with orthoses had skin lesions associated with the device.

Many surgical options have been reported for managment of CrCL disease in dogs. They can be divided into intra-articular, extracapsular, and extra-articular (osteotomies). Intra-articular methods include under-over, and over-the-top procedures (Arnoczky et al., 1979). Extracapsular methods include lateral retinacular imbrication (Flo, 1975), and fibular head advancement. Extra-articular methods include TPLO (Slocum 1993), and tibial tuberosity advancement (TTA, Montavan 2002). Some of these techniques will be explained in detail in this chapter, including the surgical planning, surgical technique, postoperative care, potential complications and long-term outcome.

The outcome after surgery is generally favourable and the most recent literature has shown a better long-term outcome for TPLO when compared to TTA and lateral fabellotibial suture (Gordon-Evans et al., 2013; Krotscheck, 2016).

EXTRACAPSULAR REPAIR FOR MANAGEMENT OF CRANIAL CRUCIATE LIGAMENT DISEASE

INTRODUCTION

Extracapsular stabilisation techniques mimic the various functions of the CrCL by placing heavy-gauge suture around the stifle joint (i.e. in an extracapsular position) in a similar orientation to the normal CrCL. The lateral fabellotibial suture (LS) is the most popular technique and has been in continuous evolution since it was first reported in the early 1970s (Johnson, 2013; Tonks et al., 2011). Despite the development in recent years of many new techniques for the management of CrCL disease, and the refinement of the dynamic stabilisation techniques, LS stabilisation is still reported to be the most commonly performed procedure by both surgery specialists and general practitioners for management of CrCL disease in small-breed dogs (<15 kg) (Comerford et al., 2013; Duerr et al., 2014).

The LS technique has always been popular for many reasons, which include its relative technical simplicity, low cost and complication rate, and the absence of catastrophic complications related to the technique itself. However, it has several limitations. The lack of true isometry of the femoral and tibial anchorage points prevents constant suture tension throughout the full range of motion of the joint, causing slackening of the suture, which often results in early fatigue and failure of the implant.

> The LS technique does not restore the normal kinematics or contact mechanics of the stifle, causing decreased range of motion and increased lateral joint compartment pressures (Chailleux et al., 2007; Tonks et al., 2010).

A growing body of evidence suggests a less successful outcome for LS surgery than for alternative techniques such as TPLO, even for small dogs (Boddeker et al., 2012; Nelson et al., 2013; Gordon-Evans et al., 2013; Berger et al., 2015).

New extracapsular techniques have been developed to overcome some of the inherent limitations of the LS technique, such as the TightRope® CCL repair (Cook et al., 2010) (Arthrex Vet Systems, Naples, USA), the Simitri Stable in Stride® extracapsular articulating implant (Barkowski and Embleton, 2016) (EAI; New Generation Devices, Glen Rock, USA) or the extracapsular bone anchor Ruby® system (Muro and Lanz, 2017) (Kyon, Switzerland). It is beyond the scope of this chapter to describe these new techniques.

The LS technique relies on the ability of the body to develop periarticular fibrosis to provide long-term joint stability, because the stability provided by the implant itself is short lived (Olmstead, 1993). Two months is enough to allow for the fibrosis to develop in most patients (Tonks et al., 2011).

Surgical recommendations for standard LS stabilisation at the time of writing of this book are described in the *Surgical technique* section.

INDICATIONS

The use of the LS technique has declined in the last 15 years, particularly in larger dogs (>15 kg) and in the referral population (Leighton, 1999; Comerford et al., 2013; Duerr et al., 2014).

Although there is no absolute contraindication to the use of LS stabilisation, the complication rate significantly increases with increasing bodyweight and decreasing age of the patient at the time of surgery (Casale and McCarthy, 2009). Furthermore, in recent years dynamic CrCL stabilisation techniques and the implants used have improved dramatically and have been adapted to their use in small breeds. There is evidence that TPLO provides a better clinical outcome than the LS technique, even in small breeds (Berger et al., 2015). For this reason, the author no longer routinely performs LS surgery in patients over 5–10 kg.

> The author still recommends the use of LS stabilisation for selected cases, particularly for smaller patients or for cases with financial constraints.

The use of an alternative extracapsular technique (i.e. TightRope®) should also be considered for large patients with increased risk of postoperative tibial fracture (i.e. due to the anxious nature of the patient and the inability of the owners to restrain it).

SURGICAL PLANNING

No preoperative planning is required for LS stabilisation other than preoperative radiographs of the affected joint.

SURGICAL TECHNIQUE

Current surgical recommendations (Tonks et al., 2011; Tobias and Johnston, 2012; Aisa et al., 2015; Witte et al., 2015) for standard LS stabilisation include the use of monofilament nylon leader line because of its adequate tensile strength and minimal elastic and plastic deformation. Alternatively, much stiffer and stronger multifilament suture material can be used, but any deviation from the quasi-isometric anchorage points reported can result in failure of the technique. Furthermore, a significantly increased infection rate has been reported for some of these materials. Ethylene oxide sterilisation preserves the physical properties and handling characteristics of monofilament nylon better than steam sterilisation. The nylon line should be secured with crimp tubes as they are significantly stronger and elongate less than knots. Two pairs of femoral and tibial anchorage points have been reported to provide the best "quasi-isometry" and can be used for extracapsular techniques. One pair connects the most caudal aspect of the lateral femoral condyle at the level of the distal pole of the fabella with the cranial or caudal wall of the extensor groove in the proximal tibia (Hulse et al., 2010a; Cinti et al., 2015). Bone tunnels or anchors are required in both sites. The current standard of care for LS surgery uses the lateral femorofabellar ligament as femoral attachment and one or two bone tunnels several millimetres caudal and proximal to the tibial attachment of the patellar ligament on the tibia. The femorofabellar ligaments are not true ligaments but the tendons of origin of the two heads of the gastrocnemius muscle. The use of the femorofabellar ligament should be favoured over the lateral fabella since it is very strong and avoids potential entrapment of the peroneal nerve or loss of tension of the suture caused by the nylon slipping off the fabella. Similar anchorage points can be used in feline patients (De Sousa et al., 2014; De Sousa et al., 2015). Multiple loop configurations have been tested to identify configurations that provide sufficient strength and minimal elongation. The use of a single or a double loop configuration on a single strand of nylon, and secured with one or two crimp tubes, is currently advised. A double-loop configuration involves passing the nylon through the anchorage points twice before securing it with one or two crimp tubes. The use of a double-loop configuration or of two crimp tubes significantly increases the ultimate strength of the construct. The double-loop configuration also significantly reduces the elongation of the nylon suture (creep). It is usually recommended to use nylon suture size in pounds (related to its strength) that is equivalent to or doubles the bodyweight of the patient in pounds, depending on the manufacturer (there is roughly 1 kg in 2 lbs). Finally, the prosthesis should always be secured at 100° of stifle flexion, with the aid of a double action crimper and applying the maximum strength of both hands. This should help ensure appropriate tension of the nylon line and the crimps securing it.

The author's preference is to place the patient in dorsal recumbency at the end of the table (Fig. 8), although lateral recumbency with the affected side on top is equally suited for this procedure. Patient draping is carried out in a standard fashion. A standard lateral parapatellar approach and identification of the lateral fabella is followed by a lateral mini- or full arthrotomy, depending on the preference of the surgeon and individual case.

The skin is incised from the proximal pole of the patella to just distal to the point of insertion of the patellar tendon on the tibial tuberosity (Fig. 9). The lateral retinacular fascia of the biceps femoris is sharply incised proximodistally and 2–3 mm lateral to the patellar tendon, from the proximal pole of the patella to the point of origin of the cranial tibial muscle. The incised lateral leaf of the retinaculum is then bluntly elevated and retracted caudally until the lateral fabella can be easily palpated. The author finds that elevating the retinaculum before incising the joint capsule facilitates its elevation and identification of the fabella (Fig. 10). The lateral fabella can now be palpated on the caudolateral aspect of the distal femur, and this can be facilitated by the use of a periosteal elevator (Fig. 11). The lateral fabella is a bony structure that can be moved very slightly and independently from the femur and must be distinguished from the more distal head of the fibula, that can also be quite prominent but moves with the tibia during stifle flexion and extension.

A mini-arthrotomy is now performed to explore the joint, assess the cruciate ligaments and menisci, and provide treatment if required (Fig. 12). Alternatively, a full arthrotomy or arthroscopy can be performed. In small dogs, the author often sharply excises the infrapatellar fat pad with a number 15 scalpel blade to improve the visualisation of intra-articular structures. The author also debrides the torn CrCL and visually inspects and probes the menisci in all patients. The use of a Beaver scalpel handle and blade is useful in very small patients when performing meniscectomies. The joint is thoroughly lavaged before the joint capsule is closed with monofilament absorbable suture in a continuous fashion.

The author does lateral sutures with a single tibial tunnel, drilling the tunnel perpendicular to the long axis of the tibia and about 2–4 mm caudal and proximal to the insertion of the patella ligament on the tibial tuberosity (Fig. 13). A 1.5 to 2.5 mm drill bit on a drill or hand chuck can be used depending on the size of the nylon needle used.

Nylon leader line (i.e. 50, 80 or 100 lbs) and crimp tubes (i.e. 10 or 12 mm) of appropriate size are now selected. In terms of nylon configuration, the author favours the use of the single-loop configuration secured with two crimp tubes if they fit between anchorage points (not often the case in smaller patients). The author used to use a double-loop and double-crimp configuration in large patients when the largest commercially available nylon was neither strong nor stiff enough. The author currently favours the tibial plateau levelling osteotomy (TPLO) technique in patients over 10 kg, except in patients with a steep tibial plateau angle (TPA), in which the cranial closing wedge osteotomy (CCWO)

technique is preferred. The swaged needle is passed through the fabellofemoral ligament in a caudodorsal to craniodistal direction and the strength of the bite is assessed by gently pulling both ends of the suture (Fig. 14). The fabellofemoral ligament is located just cranial to the fabella and can be

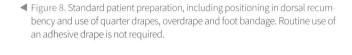

◄ Figure 8. Standard patient preparation, including positioning in dorsal recumbency and use of quarter drapes, overdrape and foot bandage. Routine use of an adhesive drape is not required.

▼ Figure 9. Initial skin incision. Note the surgeon pointing at the distal pole of the patella and proximal tibial tuberosity with the index finger and thumb, respectively.

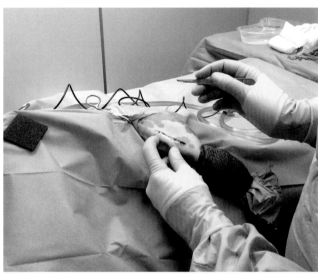

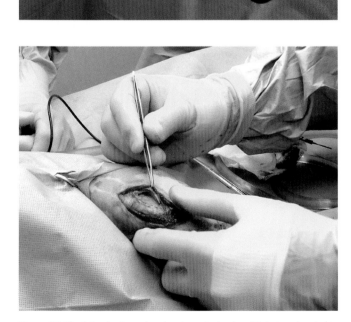

Figure 10. The lateral retinaculum has been incised and is being elevated to locate the fabella.

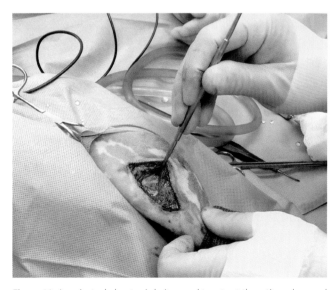

Figure 11. A periosteal elevator is being used to retract the retinaculum and locate the fabella. The blade of the elevator is located just behind (caudal to) the fabella, which can be seen located about the level of the distal pole of the patella (proximodistally).

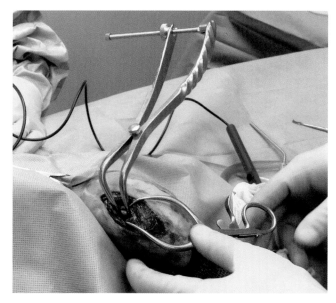

Figure 12. Note the use of a Gelpi retractor and a stifle distractor to improve the visualisation of the joint during the mini-arthrotomy. The legs of the Gelpi retractor can be secured on the patellar tendon medially and the intra-articular portion of the tendon of origin of the long digital extensor muscle laterally. The stifle distractor is introduced deep into the joint and parallel to the joint surface and then rotated 90 degrees to engage one arm on the femoral trochlear notch and another on the intercondylar area of the tibia.

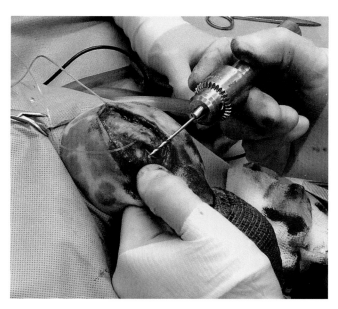

Figure 13. Thumb delineating the insertion point of the patellar ligament on the tibial tuberosity, with the tip of the drill bit resting on the lateral tibial wall at the same level. The tibial bone tunnel is drilled perpendicular to the bone axis, 2–4 mm caudal and proximal to the insertion point. Note that in this case the nylon suture has already been passed through the fabellofemoral ligament.

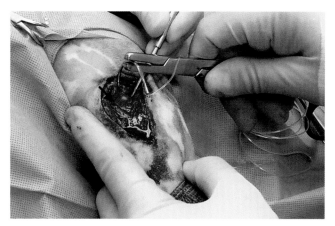

Figure 14. The periosteal elevator and needle show the most caudal and proximal aspect of the fabella respectively. The arrow indicates the location of the femorofabellar ligament and the direction that the needle must follow when it is passed through the ligament. The left index finger is on the patella. Once in this position, the point of the needle is walked cranially until it engages the femorofabellar ligament. The strength of the bite should be checked by gentle traction of the suture.

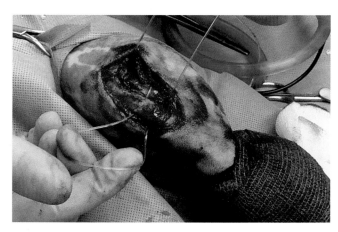

Figure 15. The nylon is passed from lateral to medial under the distal half of the patellar ligament and from medial to lateral through the tibial tunnel.

identified as the soft tissue between the bony femur and the fabella. The author sometimes uses a small Gelpi retractor to retract the lateral retinaculum and facilitate this manoeuvre. The suture is then passed under the distal half of the patellar ligament from lateral to medial and through the tibial tunnel medial to lateral (Fig. 15). All these steps can be repeated if a double-loop configuration is planned and before the suture is secured in place with one or two crimp tubes.

It is important to ensure that the stifle joint is placed at 100 degrees of flexion and with the tibia in a neutral position (avoiding cranial tibial translation and internal rotation) before the suture is tensioned and the crimp tubes are crimped (Figs. 16 and 17). The author usually tensions the nylon suture and partially crimps the tubes, then flexes and extends the joint and performs the drawer test a few times while adjusting the tension of the line as required, before fully crimping the tubes.

The suture tends to suffer some mild initial elongation and the soft tissues accommodate to the line, so further adjustments of the tension are usually required before the crimp tubes are fully tightened.

Crimping is performed in three evenly spaced locations of each crimp tube and away from its ends. Initial crimping is performed in the middle of the tube and sufficient force is applied to deform the metal enough to create adequate friction and prevent the loss of tension, but still allowing further tightening if increased tension is applied to the ends of the nylon line. Alternatively, a tensioning device can be used. The tubes are fully tightened when there is appropriate tension in the line with absence of drawer sign and the range of motion is appropriate.

The surgical site is now lavaged and closed routinely. The author tends to close with a simple continuous line of appropriately sized absorbable suture material for all planes, including the retinacular, subcutaneous and intradermal layers. Imbrication of the lateral fascia may help to further stabilise the stifle joint (Johnson, 2013). Persistence of a positive tibial compression test at a weight-bearing angle after securing the LS may be due to poor isometry of the anchorage points or insufficient tension applied to the line at the time of placement.

POSTOPERATIVE MANAGEMENT

General advice for postoperative management of orthopaedic patients applies. Specifically, strict cage or room rest and lead exercise are advised for the first 8–12 weeks postoperatively. Return to full activity should not be allowed for a minimum of 3 months.

OUTCOME

Despite the altered joint kinematics and contact mechanics after LS stabilisation, a clinical success rate between 85.7 % and 94.1 % has been reported. However, in a recent prospective force platform gait analysis study, only 40 % of dogs improved their gait, with only 14.9 % returning to normal function (Tobias and Johnston, 2012).

It is the author's experience that patients that undergo LS surgery tend to start bearing weight on the operated limb later and less consistently than those having undergone tibial osteotomy procedures. This is often the result of an excessively tight LS and tends to resolve within a week.

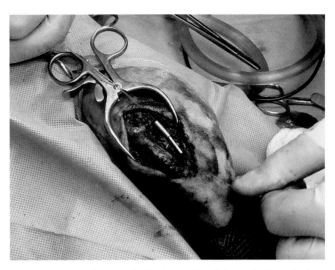

Figure 16. Suture and crimp tubes in place and ready for tensioning and crimping. Note that the joint capsule has already been closed and the lateral retinaculum is being retracted with the Gelpi retractors.

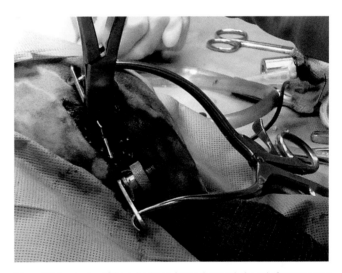

Figure 17. Tensioning of the nylon line is being done with the aid of a tensioning device in this case. Note the use of a crimper to secure the crimp tubes.

COMPLICATIONS

In a large retrospective study of 363 LS procedures, complications were recorded for 17.4 % of cases, and 7.2 % of patients required a second procedure to manage those complications. Factors significantly associated with a higher rate of complications included increasing bodyweight and young age at the time of surgery. The most common complications reported were surgical site infection and postliminary meniscal tear (Casale and McCarthy, 2009).

Postoperative loss of tension of the prostheses can occur due to suture elongation or breakage, and slippage of the suture through the crimp tube before periarticular fibrosis occurs. This can lead to recurrence of joint instability and lameness (Tonks et al., 2011).

TIBIAL TUBEROSITY ADVANCEMENT

INTRODUCTION

Tibial tuberosity advancement (TTA) was proposed in 2002 as an alternative to tibial plateau levelling osteotomy procedures (Montavon et al., 2002). According to one theoretical model, the stifle joint reaction force is approximately parallel to the patellar ligament. Tibial tuberosity advancement achieves dynamic stifle stabilisation by advancing the tibial tuberosity, thereby altering the direction of the patellar tendon (and the reaction force) until the tendon and the tibial plateau are at 90 degrees when the stifle joint angle is set at 135 degrees. This results in either a neutral or caudally directed tibiofemoral shear force during the weight-bearing phase of the gait cycle (Tepic and Montavon, 2004).

Tibial tuberosity advancement has become popular over recent years as proven by the number of TTA modifications currently present in the market (TTA rapid, TTA-2, Modified Maquet Procedure [MMP], and Porous TTA). In comparison with tibial plateau levelling osteotomy procedures, it is claimed that standard tibial tuberosity advancement and its modifications are less invasive and less technically demanding, with a reduced major complication rate. However, some reports in the current literature suggest that the complication rates are similar for tibial tuberosity advancement and tibial plateau levelling osteotomy procedures (Priddy et al., 2003; Lafaver et al., 2007). More recently, questions have been raised regarding the long-term outcome of tibial tuberosity advancement procedures and their ability to actually neutralise the tibiofemoral shear force (Murphy et al., 2014; Krotscheck et al.,2016).

INDICATIONS

The use of TTA has historically been advocated for any patient with CrCL disease; there is evidence supporting its use in dogs of any size and even in cats. Outcomes and complications are reported to be similar to the tibial plateau levelling osteotomy (TPLO) procedure, although some differences may exist in relation to infection rates, late meniscal injuries and incidence of tibial tuberosity fracture. The author would consider using this technique in dogs weighing between 20 and 50kg with favourable proximal tibial anatomy (prominent tibial crest, without excessive tibial plateau or low insertion of the patellar ligament), and particularly in cases where patellar luxation and CrCL disease are concomitant, since this can be addressed with a slight modification of the technique (tibial tuberosity transposition and advancement, TTTA).

The author's decision not to use TTA in dogs over 50kg relates to the fact that more often than not, the use of a 15 mm cage (the biggest cage commercially available) results in under-advancement in larger dogs, which may result in ongoing instability and may explain the relatively high rate (up to 50 %) of late meniscal injury reported in the literature after TTA (Murphy et al., 2014).

The author does not routinely use this technique in small dogs (<20kg) because the level of technical difficulty for this procedure increases substantially as the size of the patient decreases; in addition, small breeds commonly have an excessive tibial plateau angle which would require the use of a very large cage in relation to the plate and animal size in order to achieve a patellar tendon that is perpendicular to the tibial plateau when the stifle joint is set at 135 degrees.

Furthermore, a recent study using objective measurement of ground reaction forces as the primary outcome measure in dogs undergoing TPLO or TTA procedures showed evidence that dogs with steeper preoperative tibial plateau slopes (>27 degrees) had a better long-term outcome with TPLO compared with TTA. For this reason, the author does not recommend the use of TTA in dogs of any size where the tibial plateau angle exceeds 27 degrees (Murphy et al., 2014).

SURGICAL PLANNING

As stated in the introduction, the ultimate goal of the TTA procedure is for the patellar tendon to be perpendicular to the tibial plateau when the stifle joint is set at 135 degrees (the weight-bearing angle). It is essential to assess the required advancement and choose the appropriately sized implant (cage or wedge) to deliver and maintain this.

Several methods have been described to assess the required advancement; the three most common are the anatomical, the common tangent and the MMP methods. Current evidence suggests that the common tangent and MMP method result in less advancement than the anatomical method; however, the anatomical method requires very specific radiographic positioning (with no rotation and the stifle positioned at 135 degrees). Despite this, the anatomical method is the author's method of choice and is described here.

Standard craniocaudal and lateral radiographic projections of the affected stifle joint are obtained preoperatively to ensure no other orthopaedic conditions are present and to ascertain the required advancement. The measurement is made from the lateral view, which is centred on the stifle joint (with lack of rotation confirmed by superimposition of both femoral condyles) at an angle of 135 degrees. A correct stifle angle is crucial: if measurements are made with the stifle excessively flexed, the tibial tuberosity will be underadvanced, which may lead to residual instability and lameness, and potentially to late meniscal injury. The current recommendation from the creators of this technique is to measure with the limb in full extension.

To calculate the stifle angle following the anatomical method, it is necessary to measure the angle created by the intersection of the sagittal anatomical axes of the femur and tibia (blue line in Fig. 18). To achieve this, the full length of both the femur and tibia must be included to ensure that their long axes can be identified accurately. The femoral proximal anatomical axis is defined as the line that connects points selected 33 % and 50 % below the proximal aspect of the femoral neck in the middle of the femur (yellow line in Fig. 18). The tibial distal anatomical axis is defined as the line that connects points selected 33 % and 50 % above the distal aspect of the tibia in the middle of the tibia (green line in Fig. 18).

It is also necessary to make sure that the stifle is not subluxated ("in drawer"); if subluxation is present but not recognised, the calculated advancement will be significantly less than that actually required.

A standardised TTA transparency or computer software can be used to determine the amount of TTA required to position the patellar tendon perpendicular to the tibial plateau in a standing position; however, in the author's opinion the required advancement should be measured perpendicular to the long axis of the tibia and not the tibial plateau, since this is what actually happens when the cage is inserted at surgery (Fig. 19).

It is also necessary to assess the size of the plate needed to cover the entire extent of the tibial crest. These measurements are obtained from the lateral radiographic projection as well. Alignment of the plate guide helps to determine the number of holes (for the fork or screws) and the final plate position along the tibial crest; in some cases, it will be necessary to position the proximal end of the plate slightly caudal to ensure the distal plate holes are aligned with the cranial tibial cortex, so when the advancement is performed these distal plate holes are centred within the tibial shaft.

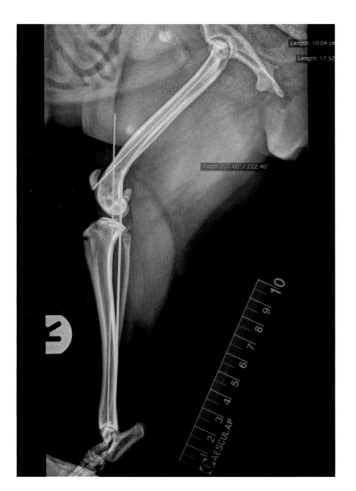

◀ Figure 18. Anatomical method used to calculate angle of stifle extension. See text to understand how to draw the different lines.

▼ Figure 19. Notice how the required advancement (double headed yellow arrow) should be measured: perpendicular to the long axis (yellow line) and not parallel to the tibial plateau (red line).

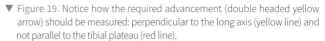

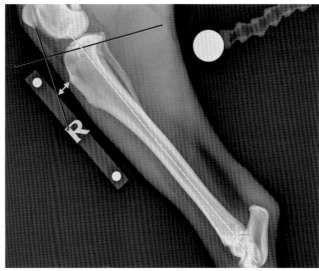

SURGICAL TECHNIQUE

The dog is positioned in dorsal recumbency. Before surgical stabilisation is performed, the stifle joint should be examined by either arthrotomy or arthroscopy to evaluate the degree of damage to the cruciate ligaments and menisci, to ensure no other conditions are present, and to treat meniscal injuries as required.

Exposure of the craniomedial aspect of the tibial crest is performed by making a skin incision relatively caudal and parallel to the long axis of the tibia that will be extended distally to the tibial diaphysis (the same distance from the end of the tibial crest as the size of the tibial crest itself). Once the subcutaneous tissue and fascia have been dissected, an incision over the cranial aspect of the insertion of the caudal belly of the sartorius muscle and the aponeurosis of the gracilis, semimembranosus, and semitendinosus muscle insertions is performed (similar to the TPLO approach, see pp. 58–59) and these structures are gently pushed caudally to expose the bone where the osteotomy will be positioned (Fig. 20). The periosteum of the tibial crest is reflected cranially to expose the cranial bone margin of the entire tibial crest; the author tends to use monopolar diathermy to achieve this.

An eight- or four-hole drill guide (Kyon) is positioned parallel to the cranial margin of the tibial crest, with the first hole aligned slightly distal to the insertion of the patellar tendon into the tibial tuberosity (Fig. 21). The number of 2.0 mm holes drilled corresponds to the plate size determined during preoperative planning. Before drilling these holes, plate orientation is checked to ensure that the distal holes are located slightly forward of the central tibial axis, so that after subsequent advancement/rotation of the tibial tuberosity, the distal screw-holes in the plate will overlie the central tibia. Sometimes, as mentioned in the planning section, it is necessary to align the proximal end of the plate slightly caudally.

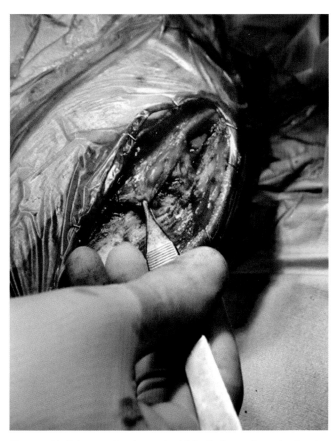

Figure 20. Medial approach to the proximal tibia. The image shows the elevation of the insertion of the caudal belly of the sartorius muscle and the aponeurosis of the gracilis, semimembranosus, and semitendinosus muscles.

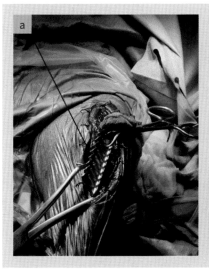
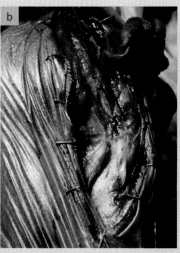

Figure 21. The drilling guide is aligned cranially and held in place using point reduction forceps distally. The k-wire is assessing bone stock through one of the drill guide holes (a). The drilled holes are reasonably cranial, as illustrated by the k-wire introduced in the most proximal hole (b).

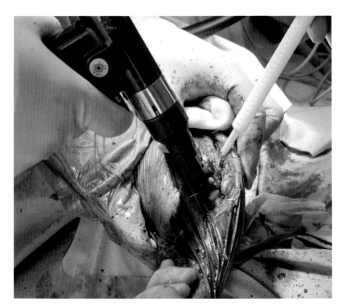

Figure 22. Initial osteotomy. Bicortical over the distal 50 % and monocortical over the proximal 50 %.

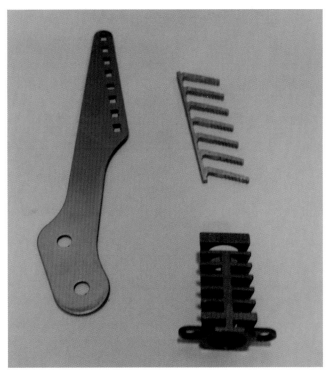

Figure 23. Tibial tuberosity advancement plate, fork and cage.

The planned osteotomy, perpendicular to the sagittal plane of the tibia, is oriented from a point immediately cranial to the medial meniscus (and cranial to the tubercle of Gerdi and the long digital extensor tendon) to the distal extent of the tibial crest. A bicortical osteotomy is performed distally, and extended only through the medial cortex for approximately one-half of the total distance proximally (Fig. 22).

A TTA tension-band plate is slightly contoured to match the shape of the tibial crest and proximal tibia. If severe contouring is required, the author prefers to rasp the bone in order to flatten it. In any case, the plate is always bent with a slight caudal rotation and distomedial bend; all bending/twisting is performed in the area between the fork and screwholes. A fork designed to fit within the tension-band plate, of the corresponding size, is locked into the plate (Fig. 23). The plate/fork combination is then secured into the tibial crest (which requires impaction of the fork with a mallet into the predrilled holes in the bone) (Fig. 24).

The remainder of the osteotomy is completed (Fig. 25) and the tibial crest, with the attached plate, is moved cranially using a spacer attached to a T-handle. In theory the spacer should correspond to the selected cage width; however, in the author's experience, it is better to use the spacer corresponding to the next cage size if possible, as this will make cage placement far easier (Fig. 26).

The depth of the bone is measured proximally, a cage of sufficient length is selected and the "ears" of the cage (screw-holes) are contoured to match the corresponding tibial surfaces (cranial ear bent downwards and caudal

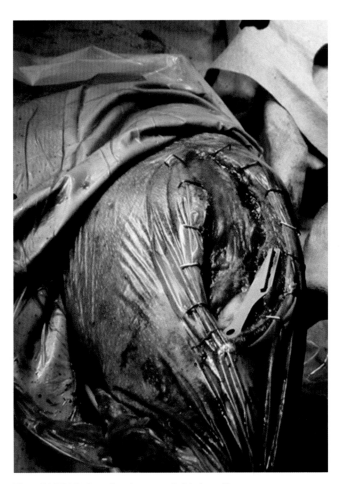

Figure 24. Tibial tuberosity advancement plate in position.

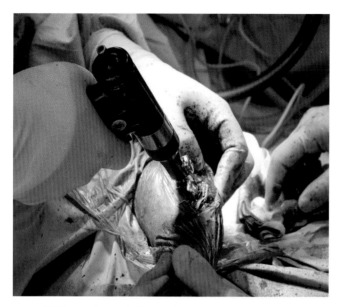

Figure 25. The osteotomy is finished proximally.

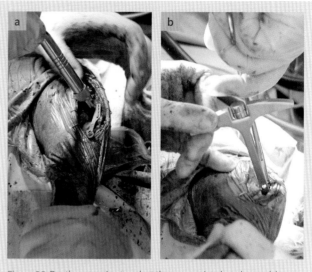

Figure 26. Depth measuring to select the appropriate length cage (a). Positioning of the spreader and cage (b).

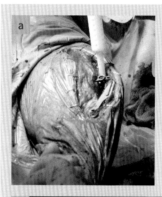

Figure 27. Cage and plate position prior to screw placement (a). Postoperative lateral radiograph showing correct plate, osteotomy and cage positioning (b).

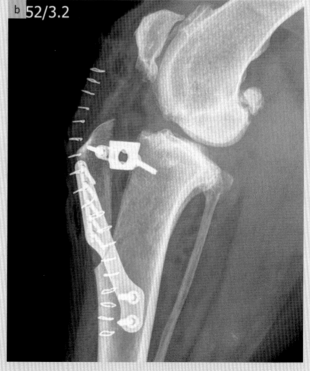

ear bent upwards). The selected cage is then placed into the osteotomy site at the proximal extent of the osteotomy (2–3 mm from the proximal tibial bone margin). It is important to check that the cranial ear is in a good position (good bone stock, and not aligned with the patellar tendon insertion). The entire tibial crest is allowed to shift a few millimetres proximally to ensure that the patellar position remains unaltered (the arc of rotation of the patellar tendon's attachment to the tibial tuberosity centred at the patella). Point reduction forceps are used to compress the distal osteotomised tibial crest to the rest of the tibia. At this stage, the plate is secured distally to the tibia with an appropriately sized screw (2.7 mm for up to five-hole plates; 3.5 mm for bigger sizes); then the cranial cage screw is secured into the tibial tuberosity in a cranioproximal direction and the caudal screw in a caudodistal direction. Finally, the distal plate screw is inserted. The limb is evaluated to confirm the absence of a positive tibial compression test. A bone graft (autologous or artificial) can be placed into the osteotomy. Closure is routine. Postoperative radiographs are always obtained to evaluate correct implant positioning (Fig. 27).

COMPLICATIONS AND LONG-TERM OUTCOME

Complications are a significant possibility. The main concerns are late meniscal injury and tibial tuberosity fracture. More often than not tibial tuberosity fractures are asymptomatic; however, sometimes they need surgical intervention. The strategy is to try to avoid their occurrence in the first instance. Narrow distal osteotomy, low cage placement and caudal placement of the plate are technical errors associated with tibial tuberosity fracture. If a fracture occurs and needs stabilisation, tension-band wiring or cranial plating have been reported to be successful.

Late meniscal injury has been reported in around 10 % of cases and it is likely to be linked to under-advancement; this illustrates the importance of good surgical planning. On the other hand, TTA seem to be associated with a reasonably low infection rate (implant removal needed in 1.3 % of cases), with very few cages reported to be removed in the literature.

They main concern currently is a suspected poor functional outcome in animals with an excessive tibial plateau angle (>27 degrees) when treated with TTA. As a rule of thumb, if the tibial tuberosity cannot be advanced by the desired amount, then TTA is probably not a suitable technique in that patient.

There are several modifications of the original TTA procedure, some of which do not use plates to stabilise the crest; these modifications are collectively known as plateless tibial tuberosity advancement (TTA rapid, MMP, Porous TTA etc.). Many of these modifications do not allow the tibial crest to "jump up" proximally since their proposed osteotomy is incomplete (attached distally). This can result in under-advancement, based on the fact that the cage is relatively more proximal in relation to the patellar tendon insertion. Furthermore, tibial diaphyseal fractures have recently been reported with plateless TTA. Tibial diaphyseal fracture is a rare occurrence with the original TTA technique.

TIBIAL PLATEAU LEVELLING OSTEOTOMY

INTRODUCTION

Rupture of the CrCL is one of the most common causes of pelvic limb lameness in the dog (Johnson et al., 1994; Aiken et al., 1995).

The CrCL is an important stabiliser of the stifle joint. It prevents hyperextension of the joint and internal rotation of the tibia, and opposes cranial tibial thrust resulting from forces generated by muscle contraction and external ground reaction forces during the weight-bearing phase, thus limiting cranial displacement of the tibia (Slocum and Devine, 1984; Jerram et al., 2005).

Diverse causal factors have been described, though it is generally accepted that CrCL rupture is primarily a degenerative phenomenon in dogs (Slocum and Devine, 1984; Vasseur, 1993; Duval et al., 1999; Wilke et al., 2005; Krayer et al., 2008).

In 1993, Slocum and Slocum proposed that the magnitude of cranial tibial thrust was a major component of instability and was related to tibial plateau angle (TPA) (Slocum and Slocum, 1993). A tibial plateau levelling osteotomy (TPLO) technique was developed to convert the cranial tibial thrust force into a joint compressive force, thus addressing this component of instability, in order to resolve pain and lameness without replacing the ligament itself. It establishes dynamic stability of the stifle and negates the requirement for passive restraint.

Warzee et al. (2001) demonstrated neutralisation of the cranial tibial thrust at a TPA of 6.5 degrees in an in vitro study. Subsequent studies have shown acceptable outcomes in patients (in vivo) with a postoperative TPA after TPLO of up to 14 degrees (Robinson et al., 2006).

> Aiming for a postoperative TPA of 4–6 degrees for dynamic stabilisation of a CrCL-deficient stifle is advised.

INDICATIONS

TPLO is generally indicated in patients with a deficient CrCL without concurrent caudal cruciate ligament disease.

TPLO is a versatile technique which is performed in dogs in dogs over 5 kg and under 100 kg (Fitzpatrick and Solano, 2010) and in small-breed dogs with a steep TPA (>30 degrees) (Witte and Scott, 2014). Reports of successful TPLO surgery performed on other species such as cats (Mindner et al., 2016) and alpaca (Smith et al., 2009) can be found in the literature.

Bilateral simultaneous TPLO surgery has been reported, with contradictory conclusions with regard to the number of postoperative complications when compared with staged procedures (Bergh et al., 2008; Fitzpatrick and Solano, 2010). It is the author's opinion and daily practice to consider the level of the patient's disability at the time of presentation before deciding whether to perform simultaneous or staged TPLO surgeries. Generally, the decision is made to perform simultaneous procedures when dogs are unable to ambulate, but other nonclinical factors (i.e. financial restrictions) are also taken into consideration.

SURGICAL PLANNING

Orthogonal stifle radiographs are taken of the affected and contralateral stifles (mediolateral and caudocranial views). Radiographic signs consistent with cranial cruciate ligament disease, such as increased opacity suggestive of stifle effusion on mediolateral radiographs (cranial displacement of the infrapatellar fat pad and caudal displacement of the subgastrocnemius fascia) and presence of osteophytes cranial to the tibial plateau at the level of insertion of the cranial cruciate ligament and at the apex of the patella, are generally seen (see Fig. 4 in *Cranial cruciate ligament disease - Clinical history, physical examination and diagnosis*, p. 43).

Mediolateral views are taken, collimated to include the stifle and hock joint. The stifle must be flexed to 90 degrees and perfect positioning is paramount for measurement of the preoperative TPA. The radiographic beam is centred in the stifle to minimise distortion. The femoral condyles should be superimposed with overlapping of the tibial intercondylar eminences, although in patients with femoral and or tibial deformities, this may not be achieved. It is important to include a device to calibrate the images when digital software is used for measurements (Fig. 28).

A line connecting the cranial and caudal aspects of the tibial plateau is drawn (tibial plateau axis). A second line dividing the intercondylar eminences and joining the centre of rotation of the talus determines the tibial long axis.

The tibial plateau angle is measured at the intersection of the tibial plateau axis and the tibial long axis with reference to a line perpendicular to the tibial long axis. It can also be determined by measuring the original angle between the two lines and subtracting 90 degrees, or with the use of a software program with digital radiography (Fig. 29).

The next step is to determine the size of the TPLO blade. Acetate templates can be overlaid on traditional radiographs, but the author prefers to use digital radiography and a TPLO measurement software program. The TPLO blade is centred at the centre of rotation of the stifle between the femoral condyles and the intercondylar eminences of the tibia (Fig. 30) to represent the circular osteotomy.

A postoperative tibial tuberosity width of >10 mm at the level of insertion of the patellar tendon is ideal (Bergh et al., 2008). In small-breed dogs, this distance should be at least 6–7 mm. Maximising the size of the blade within the mentioned recommendations for tibial tuberosity width allows the use of larger implants and minimises difficulties of implant positioning. Modifications of the centring of the TPLO blade by a few mm (i.e. caudal and/or distal centring) can be performed to allow optimal osteosynthesis with an associated distortion of the postoperative TPA and/or tibia length but a generally similar clinical outcome. Once the size of the TPLO blade has been chosen, the use of a standardised TPLO rotation chart (Table 1) or radiographic software program can

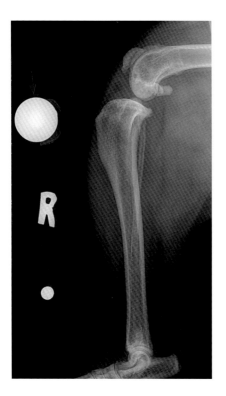

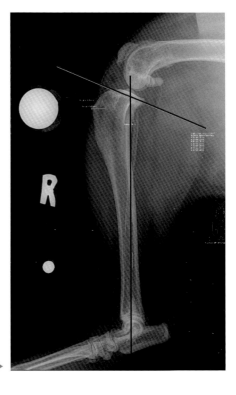

◄ Figure 28. Mediolateral radiograph of the stifle with the femur and tibia at a 90-degree angle. Collimation should include the patient's hock for measurement of the tibial plateau angle (TPA). The red arrow shows an example of a calibration device. In this case, a 20 mm sphere is placed at the same height as the patient's stifle and used to calibrate all measurements.

Figure 29. Preoperative tibial plateau axis line (red line) and tibial long axis (black line). ▶

be consulted to determine the rotation required for each preoperative TPA and blade size. TPLO blades range from 8 to 30 mm.

Preoperative measurements can facilitate intraoperative positioning of the circular osteotomy (more centred osteotomy) and reduce the chances of postoperative tibial tuberosity fractures (Collins, 2014). Two references for intraoperative landmarks are measured preoperatively. The first, A, is the distance between the insertion of the patellar tendon to the circular osteotomy, measured along a line perpendicular to the tibia. The second, B, is the distance measured along the cranioproximal border of the tibia, along a line from the insertion of the patellar tendon to the point of intersection with the circular osteotomy of the TPLO blade (Fig. 31).

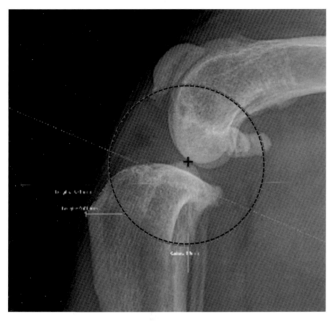

Figure 30. TPLO blade selection (red circle) using a digital template. The blade is centred at the centre of rotation of the stifle (red cross) between the intercondylar eminences and femoral condyles.

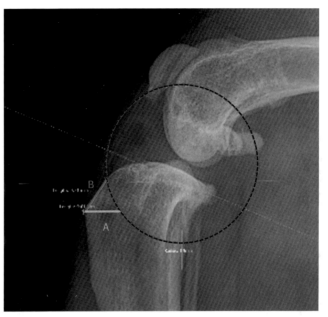

Figure 31. Presurgical measurements of distances A and B. Distance A is measured along a line perpendicular to the tibia, from the tibial tuberosity at the level of insertion of the patellar tendon to the point of intersection with the circular osteotomy of the TPLO blade. This distance has to be ideally >10 mm in large-breed dogs and a minimum of 6–8 mm in small-breed dogs. Distance B is the distance between the tibial tuberosity at the level of insertion of the patellar tendon to the most proximal aspect of the tibial plateau at the exiting level of the TPLO blade.

TABLE 1. Standardised TPLO rotation chart.

	15°	16°	17°	18°	19°	20°	21°	22°	23°	24°	25°	26°	27°
12 mm	2.0	2.2	2.4	2.6	2.9	3.1	3.3	3.5	3.7	3.9	4.1	4.3	4.5
15 mm	2.6	2.8	3.1	3.3	3.6	3.8	4.1	4.3	4.6	4.9	5.1	5.4	5.6
18 mm	3.1	3.4	3.7	4.0	4.3	4.6	4.9	5.2	5.5	5.8	6.1	6.5	6.8
21 mm	3.6	4.0	4.3	4.7	5.0	5.4	5.8	6.1	6.5	6.8	7.2	7.5	7.9
24 mm	4.1	4.5	5.0	5.4	5.8	6.2	6.6	7.0	7.4	7.8	8.2	8.6	9.0
27 mm	4.7	5.1	5.6	6.0	6.5	7.0	7.4	7.9	8.4	8.8	9.3	9.7	10.2
30 mm	5.2	5.7	6.2	6.7	7.2	7.8	8.3	8.8	9.3	9.8	10.3	10.8	11.3
	28°	29°	30°	31°	32°	33°	34°	35°	36°	37°	38°	39°	40°
12 mm	4.7	4.9	5.1	5.3	5.5	5.7	5.9	6.1	6.3	6.4	6.6	6.8	7.0
15 mm	5.9	6.1	6.4	6.6	6.9	7.1	7.4	7.6	7.9	8.1	8.4	8.6	8.8
18 mm	7.1	7.4	7.7	8.0	8.3	8.6	8.9	9.2	9.5	9.8	10.1	10.3	10.6
21 mm	8.3	8.6	9.0	9.3	9.7	10.0	10.4	10.7	11.1	11.4	11.8	12.1	12.4
24 mm	9.5	9.9	10.3	10.7	11.1	11.5	11.9	12.3	12.7	13.1	13.5	13.9	14.3
27 mm	10.6	11.1	11.6	12.0	12.5	12.9	13.4	13.8	14.3	14.7	15.2	15.6	16.1
30 mm	11.8	12.3	12.9	13.4	13.9	14.4	14.9	15.4	15.9	16.4	16.9	17.4	17.9

THE STIFLE

A template to determine the best TPLO plate size is used. Implants are generally available from 2.0 mm to broad 3.5 mm plates with their respective screws. For giant and heavy breed dogs (>60–65 kg), a cranial broad 3.5 mm locking plate and a caudal 2.7 mm DCP/LCP/SOP plate are recommended to provide additional stabilisation. The use of a locking plate and screws was reported to reduce the risk of infections in dogs >50 kg (Solano et al., 2015).

> The author recommends the general use of locking plate constructs for TPLO as locking screw fixation serves to increase stabilisation of the TPA during TPLO healing and provides improved radiographic evidence of osteotomy healing (Conkling, 2010).

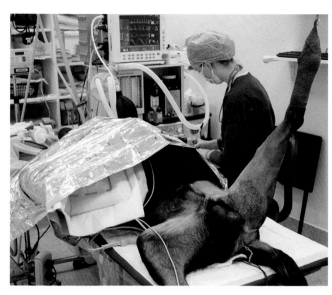

Figure 32. Patient's positioning in the theatre before draping. Hanging limb technique for surgical preparation.

SURGICAL TECHNIQUE

The author positions the dog in dorsal recumbency (Fig. 32). Following surgical preparation of the limb, standard four-quarter draping is performed and an adhesive iodine-impregnated drape is applied.

An incision is made on the craniomedial aspect of the stifle, from the cranial pole of the patella to the proximal quarter of the medial aspect of the tibia. A craniomedial parapatellar arthrotomy is performed for stifle joint exploration; alternatively, this can be done using arthroscopy. Following stifle arthrotomy, a stifle distractor is positioned between the femoral intercondylar fossa and the cranial aspect of the tibial plateau to provide optimal exposure of the joint and allow cranial subluxation of the tibia (Fig. 33). The CrCL is inspected and palpated with a meniscal probe (Fig. 34).

If substantial fraying is seen, the entire ligament is excised. The ligament is left in situ only when no grossly evident tear is visible or palpable, as it may have some function and slow the progression of osteoarthritis (Hulse, 2010b). A blunt probe is used to palpate the entire surface of the medial and

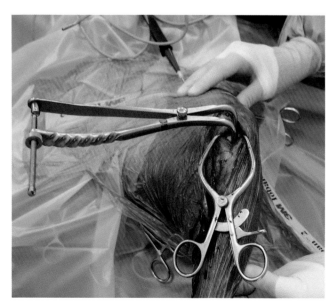

Figure 33. Intraoperative image after stifle arthrotomy with stifle distractor in place for examination of the joint.

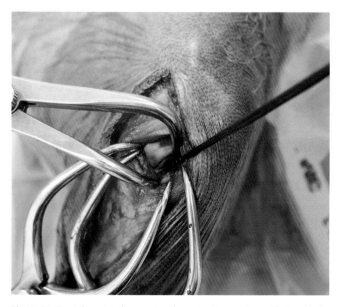

Figure 34. Cranial cruciate ligament and meniscal inspection with the aid of a meniscal probe for palpation.

lateral menisci and the tip is hooked under the caudal pole of the medial/lateral meniscus abaxial to the meniscotibial ligament and pulled cranially to assess integrity. The state of the cruciate ligament, cartilage, caudal ligament and menisci should be documented. Meniscal injuries are discussed in the *Meniscal pathology and treatment* section, pp. 71–78.

The surgical procedure is performed as described by Slocum and Slocum (1993). Subcutaneous tissues are debrided, thus exposing the pes anserinus (insertion of the sartorius, gracilis and semitendinosus muscles) on the medioproximal aspect of the tibia (Fig. 35). The pes anserinus is elevated either from proximal to distal or from distal to proximal. A tool can be slid to elevate it before transection of its aponeurosis (Fig. 36). Careful dissection is performed to expose the medial collateral ligament (Fig. 37). A 25-gauge needle is "walked" caudal to the medial collateral ligament from the proximal tibia towards the joint to determine the most proximal aspect of the tibial plateau when the needle enters the joint (Fig. 38). The use of larger needles is not recommended as meniscal injury was reported with the use of a 20-gauge needle (O'Brien and Martinez, 2009).

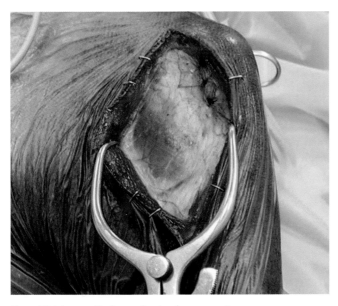

Figure 35. Intraoperative image showing the pes anserinus.

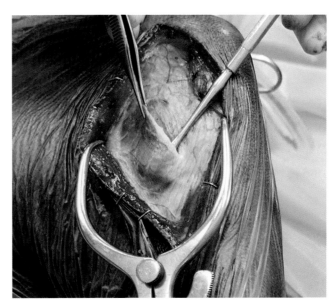

Figure 36. Elevation of the pes anserinus in a proximal to distal fashion.

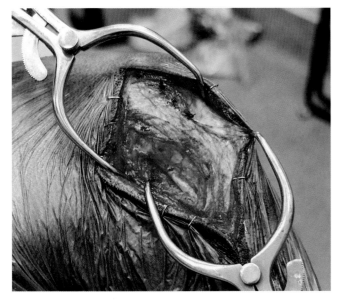

Figure 37. Exposure of the medial collateral ligament after retraction of the pes anserinus.

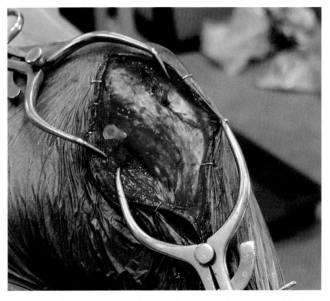

Figure 38. A 25-gauge needle is placed at the most proximal aspect of the tibial plateau, at the level of the medial collateral ligament. This is used as a reference for the placement of the proximal jig pin.

It is the author's preference to use a TPLO jig, although contradictory information has been published with regard to its benefits (Bell and Ness, 2007; Schmerbach et al., 2007). The jig helps with osteotomy orientation and reduction of the osteotomy, and facilitates limb alignment.

The most proximal pin is driven 3–4 mm from the distal joint surface and immediately caudal to the medial collateral ligament. This pin should be perpendicular to the line created by the patellar tendon (from the apex of the patella to the tibial tuberosity). This is challenging if the patient presents with a proximal tibial deformity. The proximal jig pin should be perpendicular to the sagittal plane of the tibia. An assistant is of great help to guide the primary surgeon and maintain the tibia parallel to the Table (Fig. 39). The pin is then driven into the medial cortex. Once secured, the surgeon must evaluate its location in a proximodistal and craniocaudal orientation (Fig. 40).

The chosen plate is applied to the proximal tibia close to its final location to allow the surgeon to determine the position of the distal jig pin. The distal jig pin should be away from the bottom screw of the TPLO plate to minimise the chances of creating a stress riser. With the help of the jig, the distal jig pin is driven into the centre of the tibia through the medial cortex parallel to the proximal jig pin. In patients with a significantly narrow mid-portion of the tibia, the distal jig pin may be smaller than the proximal one to minimise the risk of postoperative fractures. The position of the jig pins with respect to the tibia is then evaluated and the jig is secured. The proximal jig pin is cut short to allow circular osteotomy when needed.

Distance A is measured from the tibial tuberosity at the level of insertion of the patellar tendon and perpendicular to the crest (Fig. 41) and a mark is made on the tibia with the help of monopolar cautery (author's preference). A small incision is made caudal to the medial aspect of the patellar tendon exposing the infrapatellar bursa and the cranial edge of the proximal tibia. Distance B is measured from the tibial tuberosity at the level of insertion of the patellar tendon to the proximal aspect of the tibia at the exit level of the osteotomy and it is marked with monopolar cautery. The patellar tendon is retracted with the use of an odd-leg Gelpi retractor or a Senn retractor (Fig. 42). The TPLO saw blade is placed on the tibia such that it passes through the end of the A and B marks. Monopolar cautery is used along the edge of the TPLO saw blade to mark the circular osteotomy (Fig. 43). At this stage, the TPLO plate is applied over the tibia to evaluate the adequacy of its size and the location of the circular osteotomy before continuing (Fig. 44).

The popliteal muscle is dissected from the caudal aspect of the tibia with an initial incision followed by blunt dissection. A swab can be used to help with blunt dissection by pushing it temporarily behind the caudolateral aspect of the tibia.

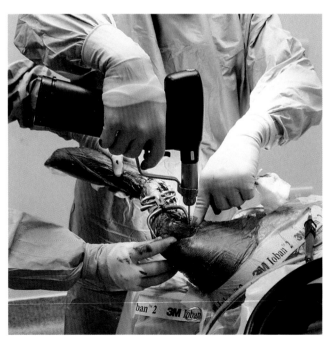

Figure 39. Intraoperative image showing the positioning of the proximal jig pin. It must be placed perpendicular to the long axis of the tibia and parallel to the stifle joint.

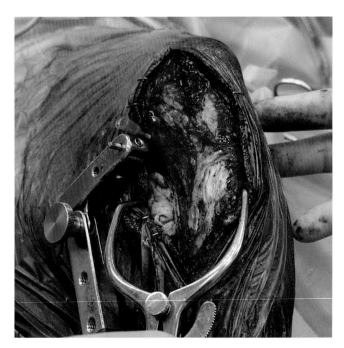

Figure 40. Close-up view of the location of the proximal jig pin, caudal and distal to the 25-gauge needle.

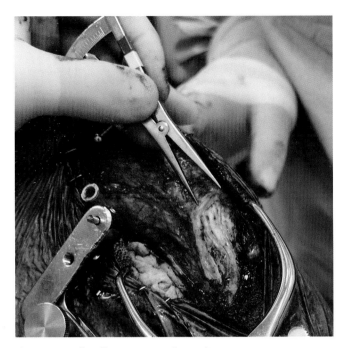

Figure 41. Use of a calliper to measure distance A.

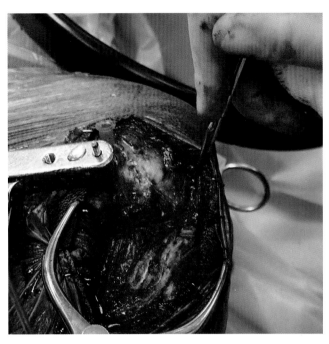

Figure 42. Retraction of the patellar tendon after performing a small arthrotomy to reveal the infrapatellar bursa.

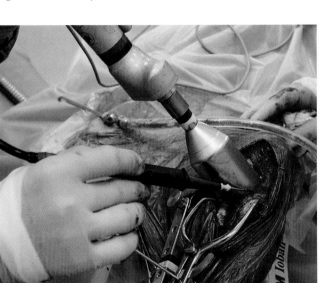

Figure 43. Monopolar cautery is used to mark the site of the circular osteotomy while the TPLO blade is positioned on the proximal tibia.

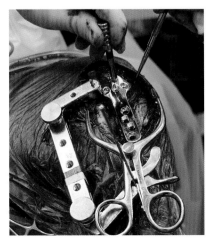

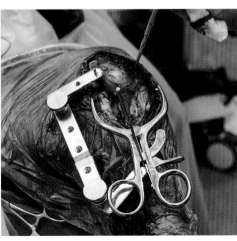

Figure 44. A TPLO plate is trialled for adequacy of size of the implant and location of the planned osteotomy before proceeding.

Several ex vivo studies (Farrell, 2011; Pozzi et al., 2011) have shown no difference in the damage to the cranial tibial or popliteal arteries with or without the use of sponges/swabs. The use of swabs has been reported to generate debris in the lavage fluid (Farrell, 2009) and therefore swabs are not recommended to be left after dissection is finished.

The circular osteotomy begins with the TPLO saw blade tilted to progress only on the caudal aspect of the osteotomy. Once an adequate indentation has been created on the tibia, the blade is tilted to begin the cranial aspect of the circular osteotomy, followed by a circular motion of the wrist to connect the cranial and caudal aspects of the osteotomy. Then, the rotation distance is marked after excision of the periosteum adjacent to the osteotomy on both tibial segments with the use of an osteotome and/or monopolar cautery (Fig. 45).

The first mark is made on the proximal segment of the tibia. The use of a calliper aids greatly in the measurement of the rotation distance before making the mark on the distal segment of the tibia. It is paramount that the marks are clearly visible. The circular osteotomy continues with the help of the assistant and the distal jig pin for orientation. The TPLO saw must be parallel to the distal jig pin and centred at the level of the proximal jig pin. The osteotomy is completed with continuous evaluation of correct orientation. It is recommended to apply substantial pressure over the saw blade to minimise heat generation (Farrell, 2011) and to notice when the far (or lateral) cortex of the tibia is crossed with the blade and the osteotomy completed. This minimises the chances of repetitive injury of the soft tissues and reduces the risk of popliteal bleeding. A rotational pin is placed in the proximal segment. The hock is flexed with the support of the primary surgeon's abdomen and a periosteal elevator is used between the proximal jig pin and the rotational pin to rotate the proximal segment (Fig. 46). Rotation is continued until the marks on the proximal and distal segments are in line. An anti-rotational Kirschner wire is driven from the tibial tuberosity proximal to the insertion of the patellar tendon and directed distal to the proximal jig pin to engage the caudal cortex of the proximal segment of the tibia (Fig. 47). The rotational pin can then be removed. The rotation marks should be evaluated and continue to be aligned.

The calcaneopatellar axis can be assessed intraoperatively using visual and palpable landmarks (lateral tip of the calcaneus, medial malleolus, central axis of the patella and fibular head) after rotation of the proximal segment. When necessary, sagittal realignment can be attained by bending the distal jig pin between the jig and the limb using plate-bending pliers.

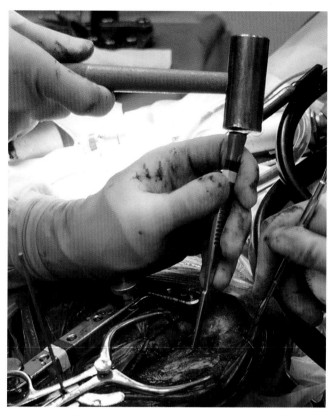

Figure 45. Use of an osteotome to mark the desired rotation distance depending on the preoperative TPA and blade size.

The TPLO plate and screws are then placed (Fig. 48). To maximise bone purchase, the screws in the proximal segment should be as caudal and proximal as possible to avoid the stifle joint. The plate is located parallel to the caudal aspect of the distal segment of the tibia. Compression at the level of the osteotomy can be applied with the help of Kern bone-holding forceps after securing the screws in the proximal segment with a partially secured (not fully tightened) single screw in the distal segment. One jaw of the Kern forceps is applied to the caudal aspect of the tibia and the other jaw to the cranial aspect of the TPLO plate. By progressively closing the Kern forceps, the distal aspect of the TPLO plate is tilted caudally and compression achieved between the segments in a craniodistal direction (Figs. 49 and 50). Alternatively, single-pointed fragment-holding forceps can be used to provide craniocaudal compression between the proximal segment and the tibial tuberosity. The cranial arm of the forceps is placed distal to the patellar tendon insertion point to avoid excessive loading of the exposed tibial tuberosity.

Abundant lavage is recommended before closure (Fig. 51). The pes anserinus is sutured first (Fig. 52) and provides cover to a portion of the plate. A tibial compression test is attempted and at this stage the results should be negative.

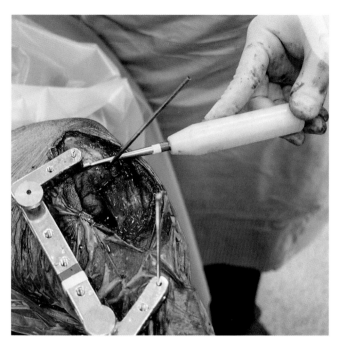

Figure 46. Use of an osteotome between the rotational pin and the proximal jig pin to facilitate rotation. The hock is flexed and secured to simplify/accelerate rotation of the proximal segment.

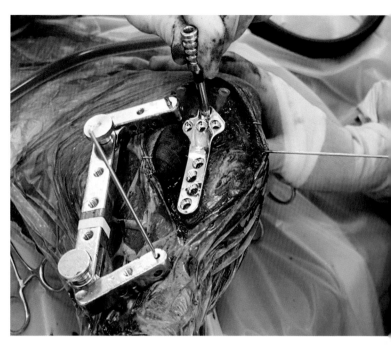

Figure 47. Anti-rotational Kirschner wire placed to temporarily secure the proximal and distal segments after rotation. The pin is placed proximal to the insertion of the patellar tendon and aiming to engage the caudal aspect of the proximal segment below the proximal jig pin.

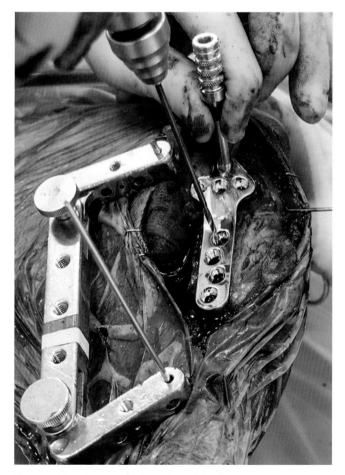

Figure 48. A broad 3.5 mm plate is used to stabilise the osteotomy.

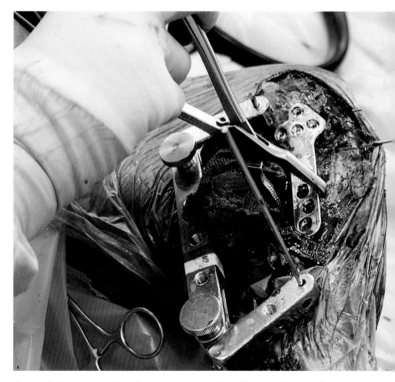

Figure 49. Kern bone-holding forceps are used in this patient to achieve additional compression between proximal and distal segments. After securing the proximal segment with locking screws, the only screw partially tightened in the distal segment behaves as a hinge. One jaw of the Kern forceps is placed on the caudal tibia distal to the screw in the distal segment, the second jaw is placed on the cranial aspect of the plate at the same level. By closing the jaws of the bone-holding forceps, compression is achieved and the distal aspect of the plate is tilted caudally.

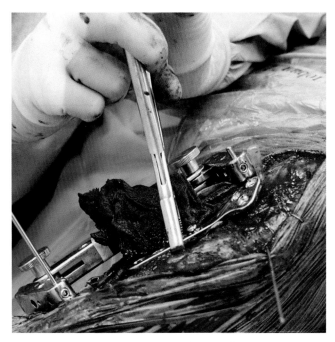

Figure 50. Additional view of the location of the Kern forceps to achieve compression at the level of the TPLO osteotomy.

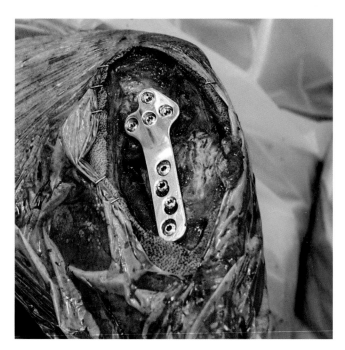

Figure 51. Four locking 3.5 mm screws have been applied to the proximal segment. Two locking 3.5 mm screws and two non-locking 3.5 mm screws have been applied to the distal segment to secure the osteotomy after rotation.

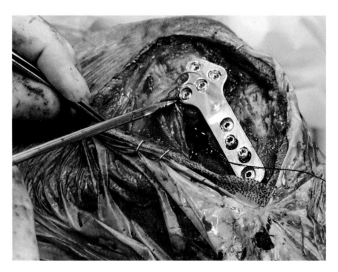

Figure 52. Closure is performed; the pes anserinus is sutured in as physiological a position as possible. This should cover a substantial portion of the TPLO plate.

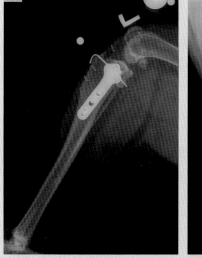
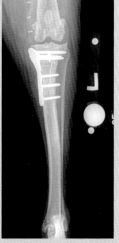

Figure 53. Postoperative mediolateral (a) and caudocranial (b) radiographs immediately after a TPLO with an optimal TPA. The antirotational K-wire was left in situ. Note the perpendicular orientation of the TPLO cut on the caudocranial view, good interfragmentary compression and plate location.

On rare occasions, with patients that underwent acute traumatic full rupture of the cranial cruciate ligament, additional stabilisation (i.e. an extracapsular technique) may be required.

The rest of the surgical wound is closed as per routine in three layers. Postoperative orthogonal radiographs are taken. Again, the radiographs should be as perfect as possible to provide the most accurate postoperative TPA measurement (Fig. 53).

POSTOPERATIVE MANAGEMENT

Perioperative antibiotic therapy is given to all patients and discontinued at the end of the surgical procedure. Heavy dogs have a higher risk of postoperative infection after TPLO (Fitzpatrick and Solano, 2010; Solano et al., 2015).

In dogs over 50 kg, a short course of broad-spectrum antibiotics (cephalexin twice a day PO for 10–14 days) is recommended. An improvement in our ability to provide more stable constructs after TPLO in heavy dogs in the future could modify this recommendation. Oral NSAIDs are provided for 14 days. The limb is not usually bandaged and it is recommended that cryotherapy is applied every 4–6 h for the first 72 h after surgery.

Strict rest is prescribed for 6 weeks (confinement in a big cage or small room). No jumping, running, off-lead exercise, walking on slippery surfaces or up and down steps or stairs is allowed. The patient can go outside on the lead for 10 minutes 3–4 times a day for toilet purposes. The skin sutures or staples are removed after 12 days. Follow-up radiographs are taken after 6 weeks under heavy sedation. Provided there is evidence of advanced healing and no implant-related issues, lead exercise can be increased by 5 minutes per walk on a weekly basis over a 4-week period, followed by slow reintroduction of off-lead exercise over an additional 4-week period. Physiotherapy has shown benefits after TPLO (Monk et al., 2006) and can be considered after the 6-week follow-up visit.

OUTCOME
The outcome after a TPLO is generally favourable and compares positively with objective long-term data when compared to tibial tuberosity advancement (TTA) and lateral fabellotibial suture (Gordon-Evans et al., 2013; Krotscheck, 2016 et al.). TPLO resulted in operated limb function that was similar to the control population by 6–12 months postoperatively at the walk and the trot in the study by Krotscheck et al. (2016). Owner satisfaction for dogs after TPLO has been reported to be as high as 93 % (Gordon-Evans et al., 2013).

COMPLICATIONS
The complication rate varies between studies with values between 11.4 and 34 % (Pachiana et al., 2003; Priddy et al., 2003; Fitzpatrick and Solano, 2010; Bergh and Peirone, 2012; Coletti et al., 2014) and is similar to other osteotomy procedures (Oxley et al., 2013b). Swelling, bruising, and seroma formation may occur in the short- or intermediate-term after surgery. Low re-operation rates have been reported to be between 4.2–6.6 % (Fitzpatrick and Solano, 2010; Gatineau et al., 2011; Oxley et al., 2013b; Coletti et al., 2014; Cosenza et al., 2015).

Infection, with rates of 1–14 % (Pachiana et al., 2003; Priddy et al., 2003; Corr and Brown, 2007; Fitzpatrick and

Solano, 2010), and late/subsequent meniscal injury, with rates of 0.7–4.3 % (Pachiana et al., 2003; Carey et al., 2005; Duerr et al., 2008; Cook et al., 2010; Fitzpatrick and Solano, 2010; Gatineau et al., 2011), are among the most relevant postoperative complications. Implant removal due to long-term infection has been reported in 7.4 % of cases with *Staphyloccoccus* spp. being the most common bacteria (Gallagher and Mertens, 2012).

Other complications such as medial patellar luxation, tibial tuberosity fracture, patellar fracture, patellar tendonitis, pivot shift, and fibular fracture have been reported after TPLO (Bergh et al., 2008; Tuttle and Manley, 2009; Gatineau et al., 2011; Rutherford et al., 2012).

In a systematic review of the literature by Bergh and Peirone (2012), the proposed risk factors for complications after TPLO were: a complete preoperative rupture of the CrCL; performing a parapatellar arthrotomy; increased patient age and bodyweight; the Rottweiler breed; single-session bilateral TPLO surgical procedures; absence of jig use; a high preoperative tibial plateau angle; medial meniscectomy; the osteotomy position; a thin craniocaudal crest width; and the surgeon's inexperience.

CRANIAL CLOSING WEDGE OSTEOTOMY

INTRODUCTION
Cranial closing wedge osteotomy (CCWO) was the first dynamic stabilisation technique developed and described for treatment of CrCL disease in dogs. This technique was initially described by Slocum in 1984 and included lateral advancement of the biceps femoris muscle to prevent cranial drawer displacement. Nowadays, advancement of the biceps femoris muscle is no longer performed.

> Dynamic stabilisation techniques such as CCWO are designed to neutralise the cranial tibial thrust force.

These techniques do not repair or replace the ruptured or diseased cranial cruciate ligament, but aim to neutralise the cranial tibial thrust by levelling the tibial plateau to the 4- to 6-degree angle required to achieve active stifle stabilisation.

With the CCWO technique, levelling of the tibial plateau is achieved by removing a wedge of bone cranially, which, in principle, shortens the tibia cranially.

Indications

CCWO is generally indicated in any patient with CrCL disease; there is evidence supporting its use in dogs ranging from 20–60 kg, with outcomes and complications similar to TPLO (Oxley et al., 2013). The author mainly uses CCWO in small dogs (5–20 kg) since the implant size (and therefore the stability of the construct) can be maximised. In addition, excessive tibial plateau angle is common in small breeds, and does not allow full stabilisation with TTA procedures or requires major rotation of the osteotomised fragment during TPLO, which could lead to loss of the caudal buttress for the tibial tuberosity, theoretically predisposing to tibial tuberosity fractures. An excessive tibial plateau angle is often associated with tibial ante-curvatum, which is also resolved when performing a CCWO. CCWO can also be used in cases of CrCL disease in immature patients, since it can be performed in young dogs prior to closure of the proximal tibial physis, while the author does not recommend TPLO or TTA procedures for dogs under 8–9 months.

SURGICAL PLANNING

First of all, the tibial plateau angle must be calculated. To do so, a medial-lateral radiographic view of the stifle and tibia including the hock is used.

> In this medial-lateral view, the stifle and hock joint should be flexed at 90 degrees and the tibia should not be rotated.

A line connecting the cranial and caudal aspects of the tibial plateau is drawn (tibial plateau axis). A second line dividing the intercondylar tubercles (also known as eminences) and joining the centre of rotation of the talus determines the tibial long axis. The tibial plateau angle is measured at the intersection of the tibial plateau axis and the tibial long axis with reference to a line perpendicular to the tibial long axis. It can also be determined by measuring the original angle between the two lines and subtracting 90 degrees (Fig. 54).

Once the tibial plateau angle (TPA) has been calculated, a wedge must be drawn in the shape of an isosceles triangle, in a position as proximal as possible while preserving sufficient bone stock for plate fixation and cerclage placement and at an adequate distance distal to the tibial tuberosity.

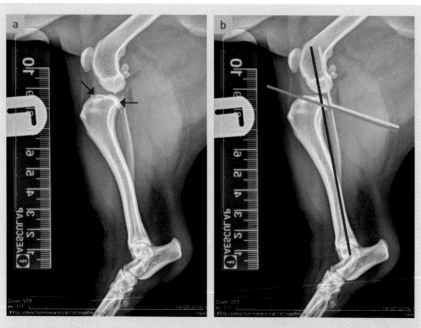

Figure 54. The yellow arrows represent both ends of the tibial long axis, while the red arrows represent the most cranial and caudal points of the tibial plateau axis (a). The tibial long axis is represented by the red line and the tibial plateau axis is represented by the blue line. The tibial plateau angle is determined by measuring the yellow angle and subtracting 90 degrees (b).

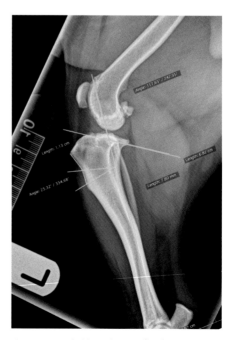

Figure 55. Medial-lateral view of a planned cranial closing wedge osteotomy. The surgeon must calculate the distance from the tibial tuberosity to the beginning of the wedge, together with the distance between the proximal and distal aspects of the wedge.

The distance from the tibial tuberosity should be a minimum of 6–7 mm in dogs weighing under 20 kg, and a minimum of 10 mm for heavier dogs (Fig. 55). The distance between the proximal and distal aspects of the wedge should also be measured.

The shape of the wedge is of paramount importance to achieve the desired postoperative tibial plateau angle. With a wedge in the shape of an isosceles triangle and maintaining a caudal cortical hinge, the planned wedge angle is usually the TPA minus 5 degrees. For example, for a 26-degree TPA, a 21-degree wedge should be drawn. However, as the TPA increases, the increasingly larger the wedge angle should be. Oxley et al. created the following table to help with this issue (Table 1).

TABLE 1. Tibial plateau angles and their corresponding wedge angle for CCWO.

TPA	Wedge angle
<20	TPA - 5
21-25	TPA- 4
26-30	TPA- 3
31-35	TPA- 2

SURGICAL TECHNIQUE

The author normally initially positions the dog in dorsal recumbency, with the contralateral hindlimb loosely tied in order to prevent it from falling towards the surgical site when rotating the dog to place the affected side adjacent to the surgical table. The author's preference is to perform the medial subpatellar arthrotomy from a cranial approach (Fig. 56).

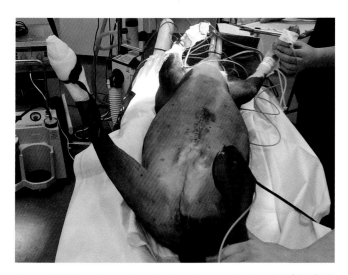

Figure 56. Initial position on the table. Note the rope placed on the left hindlimb to prevent it from moving towards the affected limb when the animal is rotated into right lateral recumbency.

Following surgical preparation of the limb, standard four-quarter draping is performed and an adhesive iodine-impregnated drape is applied. A standard medial approach to the stifle and proximal 1/3 of the tibia is then used. A craniomedial mini-arthrotomy is performed in order to confirm the presence of CrCL disease and treat meniscal injuries as required. Once the joint has been examined, the mini-arthrotomy is closed in one layer, incorporating the joint capsule and fascia lata with 2-0 or 0 polydioxanone (PDS) suture thread, depending on the dog's size and capsular thickening. At this stage, the dog is rotated so that the affected limb is adjacent to the surgery table.

The pes anserinus is elevated carefully using both sharp and blunt dissection until the medial collateral ligament is identified.

> It is a good idea to place a small orange needle in the joint to have a reference of how proximal the plate can be positioned.

The osteotomy site is identified by making measurements from the tibial tuberosity. The site of the distal osteotomy line is normally located proximal to the distal aspect of the tibial crest (Figs. 57 and 58). The proximal and distal starting points of the wedge are marked on the cranial aspect of the tibia with monopolar electrocautery. The popliteal muscle, which is located caudally, is carefully elevated using both sharp and blunt dissection in order to reveal the caudal aspect of the tibia, where the two osteotomy lines will converge to create the wedge. A small Hohman retractor is carefully placed there.

This converging point is a key aspect of the procedure, particularly if the intention is to preserve a cortical hinge that will make the procedure far easier and the construct more stable. The converging point should be located 1–2 mm cranial to the caudal aspect of the tibia. If it is located too close to it, the tibia will fracture before the wedge osteotomy is completed, while if it is located too far, the caudal aspects of the osteotomy site will contact before the cranial aspects, resulting in breakage of the cerclage wire, fracture at the drill holes, or premature fracture of the caudal cortex.

Once the wedge is marked on the medial aspect of the tibia using electrocautery, lateral subperiosteal elevation of the tibialis cranialis muscle is performed from a point 3 mm proximal to the proximal starting point of the wedge to a point 3 mm distal to the distal starting point of the wedge and a

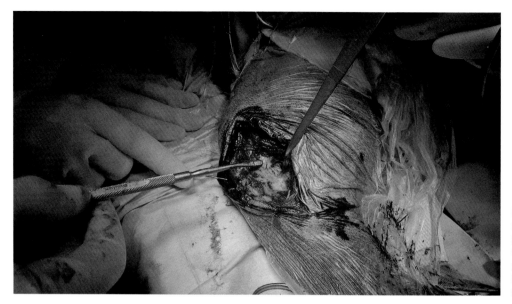

Figure 57. Intraoperative view of the medial aspect of the proximal tibia. The periosteal elevator is pointing at the medial collateral ligament. The popliteal muscle has been partially elevated and a Hohman retractor is placed caudally to allow full view of the caudal tibial cortex.

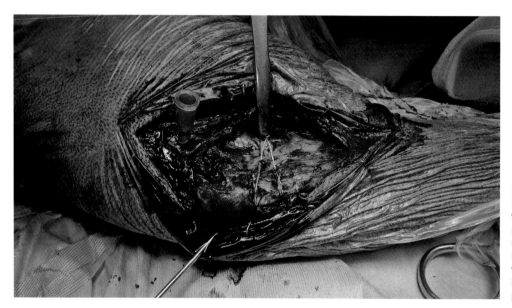

Figure 58. Intraoperative view of the medial aspect of the proximal tibia. The wedge is scored on the bone. The pin is pointing at the tibial tuberosity, where references are taken to mark the proximal and distal starting points of the wedge. Note the orange needle placed in the joint to ensure the plate is not placed too proximal.

moistened swab is placed. Before performing the osteotomy, it is best to check that the chosen plate fits comfortably (not too proximal or hanging caudally, with enough space to drill the cerclage holes).

The osteotomy is then performed with a sagittal oscillating saw, trying to preserve a small "hinge" of caudomedial cortex. At this stage, 1.1 mm or 1.5 mm drill holes are created and positioned cranially immediately proximal and distal to the osteotomy surfaces (2–3 mm away). Whenever possible, a 1.5 mm hole should be drilled and 1.2 mm cerclage wire used; 1.1 mm drill holes and 1.0 mm cerclage wires should only be used in dogs weighing less than 10–15 kg. The moistened gauze is removed and the cerclage wire is passed from medial to lateral through the proximal hole, and from lateral to medial through the distal hole. Passing the cerclage wire from lateral to medial through the distal hole can be tricky; it is best to ask an assistant to pass a small hypodermic needle from medial to lateral to aid with the location of the distal hole (Fig. 59).

Once the cerclage wire has been passed through the holes, it is tightened from medial with a single twist. It is important to remember that traction must be applied while twisting to ensure the cerclage is twisted properly. It is crucial to monitor that the wedge is closing when tension is felt. If no movement is observed, stop, replace the moist gauze and using the oscillating saw "nibble" some more bone at

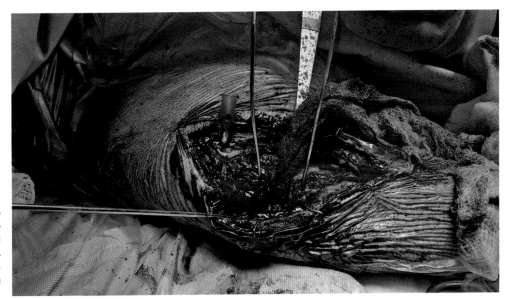

Figure 59. Intraoperative view of the medial aspect of the proximal tibia. The wedge osteotomy has been performed and the wedge has been removed. Holes have been drilled adjacent to the osteotomy site and the cerclage wire has been passed through them.

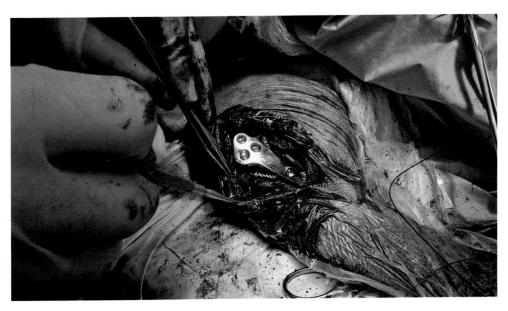

Figure 60. Intraoperative view of the medial aspect of the proximal tibia. The wedge osteotomy has been closed by twisting the wire, a broad 3.5 TPLO locking plate has been placed and the cerclage wire has been bent and placed next to the plate.

the converging point to weaken the caudal hinge. Once the wedge osteotomy is closed, the plate and screws are placed. The author's implant of choice is a TPLO locking plate (2.4 mm, 2.7 mm, 3.5 mm and 3.5 mm broad depending on the bone shape and size).

> The surgeon should not attempt to contour the TPLO locking plate, even if the proximal aspect of the plate is clearly lifting from the bone (since all the proximal screws are locking).

The first screw that should be placed is the proximal screw of the distal fragment. This frictional screw should be placed without fully tightening it, only enough to help position the plate. It is best to ask an assistant to hold the plate in position while placing two of the proximal fragment locking screws before fully tightening the compression screw. Once this is done, a locking screw is placed in the distal fragment; the rest of the screws are then placed. The cerclage wire is cut and bent at this stage and positioned parallel to the plate (Fig. 60).

Routine layered closure is performed after lavage and a sterile adhesive dressing is applied for 48 hours. Postoperative radiographs are taken in all cases to evaluate the achieved TPA and to ensure no mistakes have been made (Fig. 61).

POSTOPERATIVE MANAGEMENT

The administration of prophylactic postoperative antibiotics is a controversial issue. The author only uses perioperative antibiotics and nothing after surgery. A study evaluating TPLO found that postoperative antibiotics decrease the rate of surgical site infection (Fitzpatrick and Solano, 2010). In the author's opinion, their use should only be considered in heavy dogs (> 35 kg).

Strict rest is prescribed for 6 weeks (confinement in a big cage or small room). No jumping, running, walking on slippery surfaces and off-lead exercise, or climbing steps or stairs is allowed. The patient can go outside on the lead for 10 minutes 3–4 times a day for toilet purposes. The skin sutures or staples are removed after 12 days.

Follow-up radiographs are taken after 6 weeks under heavy sedation. Provided there is evidence of advanced healing and no implant-related issues, lead exercise can be increased by 5 minutes per walk on a weekly basis over a 4-week period, followed by slow reintroduction of off-lead exercise over an additional 4-week period. Physiotherapy can be considered after the 6-week follow-up visit.

OUTCOME

Osteoarthritis will progress; this may or may not cause problems in the future. Prognosis is good to excellent with proper postoperative care and confinement.

COMPLICATIONS

In the most recent study evaluating CCWO (Oxley, 2012), major complications occurred in 9.5 % of the cases, although reoperation rates were as low as 5.4 %. In the same study, the major complication rate for TPLO was 7.2 %, with a reoperation rate of 6.1 %.

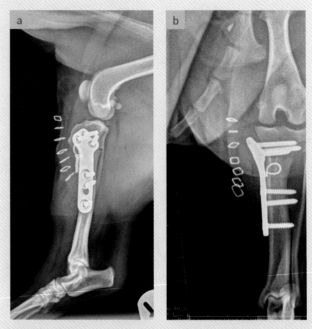

Figure 61. Medial-lateral (a) and caudal-cranial (b) postoperative radiographs of a CTWO. The postoperative tibial plateau angle was 6⁰ in this case. A 2.7 mm TPLO locking plate was used for this dog.

Most of the complications encountered were late meniscal injury requiring arthrotomy and septic arthritis, which was managed medically.

Historically, implant-related issues such as loosening and failure were commonly reported in association with this technique (Kuan et al., 2009; Corr and Brown, 20075). However, in the author's experience, such issues are not seen with the use of locking implants.

MENISCAL PATHOLOGY AND TREATMENT

INTRODUCTION

The menisci play important roles in the canine and feline stifle. They allow load transmission to be performed in an inhomogenous (varies by location) and anisotropic (direction-dependent) fashion meaning they have excellent mechanical properties. Their shock absorption properties are related to their ability to behave as a biphasic medium, which results in viscoelasticity. The menisci improve stifle joint stability by improving the congruity of the femoral condyles, thus working as a secondary stabiliser of the stifle. Another remarkable function of the menisci is the lubrication of the stifle by creation of a fluid film by the extrusion of water during loading of the joint (Tobias, 2012).

Evaluation of meniscal integrity is most commonly performed in patients with suspected CrCL disease, as up to 84.6 % of dogs with CrCL disease are reported to have concurrent meniscal injury (McCready and Ness, 2016).

Although meniscal injury in isolation has been reported in dogs (Hulse and Johnson, 1998; Langley-Hobbs, 2001; Williams, 2010), it remains as a rare event since it is usually secondary to the stifle instability that results from CrCL failure (Flo, 1993; Johnson et al., 2004).

The incidence of injury of the medial meniscus has been reported to be higher than of the lateral meniscus (McCready and Ness, 2016). It has been hypothesised that the higher incidence of tears in the medial meniscus is related to its anatomical particularities. The mobility of the medial meniscus is limited by its more extensive coronal ligament attachment to the joint capsule, and its attachment to the medial collateral ligament (Carpenter and Cooper, 2000) (Fig. 1).

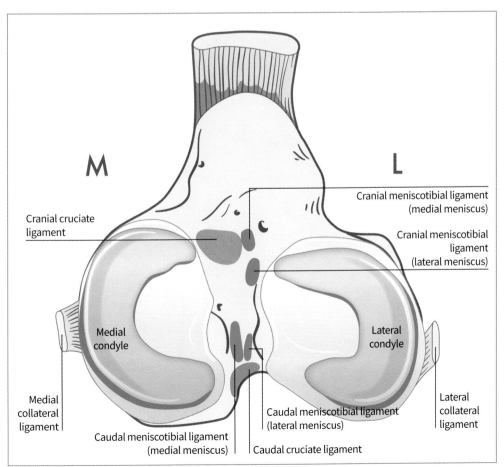

Figure 1. Anatomical diagram of the meniscotibial ligament and cranial and caudal cruciate ligaments attachments on the canine tibia. Adapted from: Tobias KM, Johnston SA, *Veterinary Surgery: Small Animal*, 2nd ed. (2017).

Complete rupture of the CrCL, longer duration of lameness and higher bodyweight have been proposed as risk factors of meniscal injury in patients presenting with CrCL disease (Fitzpatrick and Solano, 2010; Hayes et al., 2010).

> The incidence of clinically apparent subsequent/late meniscal injury (SMI) after cranial cruciate ligament repair varies depending on the surgical technique and has been reported to be from 1–27.8 % (McCready and Ness, 2016).

A higher incidence is reported in studies where TTA was used for dynamic stabilisation of the affected stifle (McCready and Ness, 2016).

Meniscal injury patterns should be recorded during surgical examination, and are classified as vertical longitudinal tear, "bucket" handle tear (vertical longitudinal tear with axial portion displaced), flap tear, radial tear, horizontal tear, complex tears and degenerative tears (Whitney, 2003) (Fig. 2). The most common reported meniscal tears in one study of dogs with concurrent cruciate ligament disease were "bucket" handle tears involving the caudal pole of the medial meniscus, which occurred in 57 % of cases (Ralphs and Whitney, 2002).

Medial meniscal release (MMR) has been recommended based on its putative biomechanical advantage, the aim being to mitigate subsequent meniscal injury (SMI) (Slocum and Devine, 1998; Pacchiana, 2003), but this is not completely protective (Thieman et al., 2006; Fitzpatrick and Solano, 2010) and results in exacerbation of medial joint compartment loading. Meniscal release is equivalent to caudal hemimeniscectomy with regard to meniscal function, further supporting the importance of an intact functional unit formed by the meniscal ligaments and the peripheral rim (Pozzi et al., 2008; Kim et al., 2009). Adequate meniscal inspection with the use of a meniscal probe together with palpation, and/or the use of magnification and light when arthroscopic inspection is performed, have been shown to increase sensitivity for the detection of meniscal injuries (Pozzi et al., 2008).

DIAGNOSIS OF MENISCAL INJURIES

Patients presenting with concurrent CrCL disease and meniscal injury are generally lame. A meniscal click has been reported in some patients with concurrent cruciate disease and meniscal injury during flexion/extension of the affected stifle. The sensitivity of an audible "clicking" sound during cranial drawer and tibial compression tests was reported as 58 % (Neal et al., 2015) and with a modified tibial compression test with axial loading up to 63–77 % (Valen, 2017).

> Damage to the menisci cannot reliably be confirmed on physical examination alone (Flo, 1993). Arthroscopy and meniscal probing are currently the gold standard for the diagnosis of meniscal injuries in the dog (Dillon, 2014).

For cases with clinical SMI after TPLO, the time frame has been reported as 125 days (range 14–450 days) (Fitzpatrick and Solano, 2010).

Classically, patients with a clinical SMI develop an acute onset of severe lameness which does not resolve with rest and administration of NSAIDs. On examination, dogs with SMI tend to show signs of pain associated with stifle flexion, digital pressure over the caudomedial aspect of the stifle and pain when the stifle is flexed while applying simultaneous internal/external rotation of the tibia. The diagnosis can be confirmed during arthrotomy or arthroscopic examination of the affected stifle (Fig. 3). Detection of meniscal tears by arthroscopy appears superior to arthrotomy in retrospective (Plesman et al., 2013) and cadaveric studies (Pozzi et al., 2008). (Fig. 4).

Other imaging modalities have been reported for detection of meniscal injuries. High-field magnetic resonance imaging (MRI) has a higher sensitivity (75–100 %) and specificity (94–100 %) than low-field MRI (sensitivity 64–100 %, specificity 89–94 %) for detection of meniscal injuries (Gonzalo-Orden et al., 2001; Blond et al., 2008; Barrett et al., 2009; Böttcher et al., 2010; Harper et al., 2011; Olive et al., 2014; Taylor-Brown et al., 2014) and particular criteria have been postulated for accurate detection (Barret et al., 2009) (Figs. 5 and 6). MRI of the affected stifle can be performed in patients that do not have stainless-steel metal implants (i.e. titanium implants); stainless-steel implants (standard TPLO plates and screws) would create a regional magnetic artefact limiting the diagnostic value. MRI should facilitate the detection of horizontal

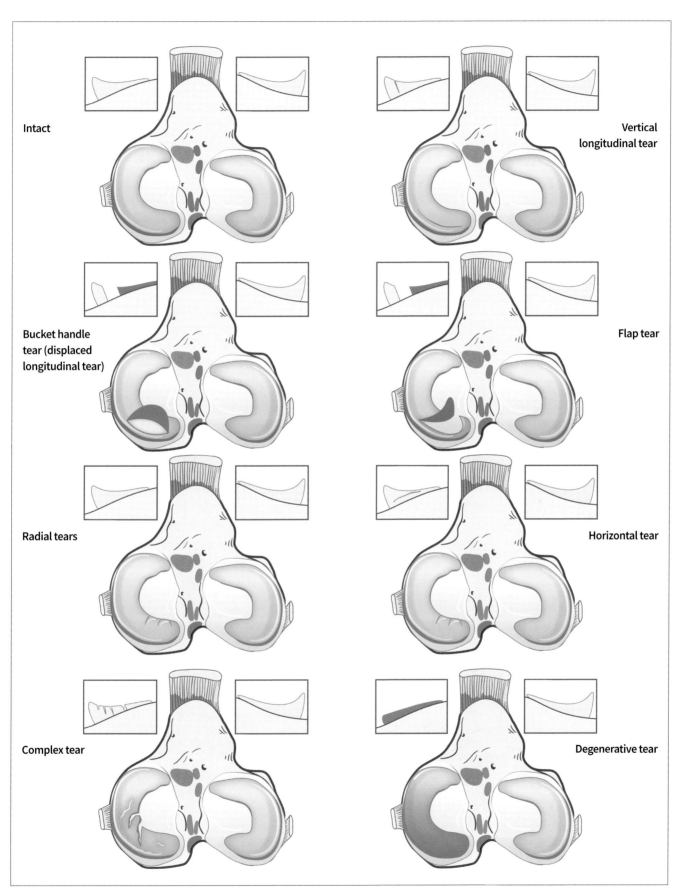

Intact

Vertical longitudinal tear

Bucket handle tear (displaced longitudinal tear)

Flap tear

Radial tears

Horizontal tear

Complex tear

Degenerative tear

Figure 2. Morphology of meniscal tears. Adapted from: Tobias KM, Johnston SA, *Veterinary Surgery: Small Animal*, 2nd ed. (2017).

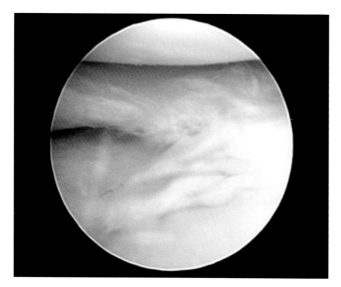

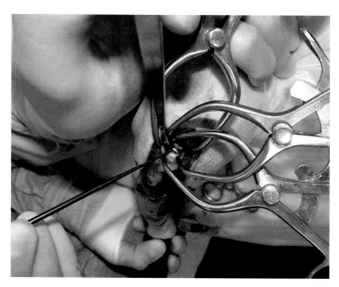

Figure 3. Arthroscopic examination of a stifle with cranial cruciate ligament disease and concurrent meniscal injury.

Figure 4. Intraoperative picture showing the use of a meniscal probe for inspection to reveal a "bucket handle" tear of the medial meniscus.

meniscal tears in menisci that may appear intact during arthrotomy/arthroscopy assisted examination; however, the clinical relevance of these remains unknown. Cost and availability limits the regular clinical use of high-field MRI for the diagnosis of meniscal injuries. Ultrasonography for the diagnosis of meniscal injuries is operator and equipment-dependent (Mahn et al., 2005; Arnault et al., 2009). Computed tomography (CT) arthrogram has been shown to be a reliable method for identifying simulated meniscal injuries in a cadaveric study (Tivers et al., 2009)

SURGICAL TECHNIQUES

MENISCAL INSPECTION: MEDIAL AND LATERAL ARTHROTOMY

This section covers the surgical management of meniscal injuries by stifle arthrotomy.

The author positions the dog in dorsal recumbency. Following surgical preparation of the limb, standard four-quarter draping is performed and an adhesive iodine-impregnated drape is applied (see Fig. 34 in *Tibial plateau levelling osteotomy - Surgical technique*, p. 58).

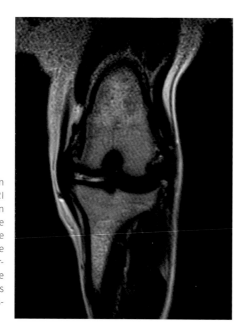

Figure 5. Proton density (PD) MRI sequence of a stifle in a craniocaudal plane with cranial cruciate ligament disease demonstrating hyperintense signal on the medial meniscus suggestive of meniscal tear.

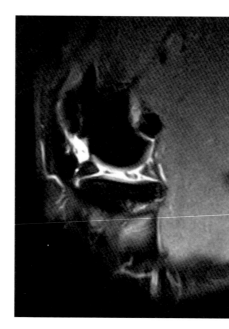

Figure 6. Proton density (PD) MRI sequence of a stifle in a sagittal plane with cranial cruciate ligament disease demonstrating hyperintense signal on the medial meniscus suggestive of meniscal tear.

A medial/lateral parapatellar approach to the stifle is the author's preference for meniscal inspection. A parapatellar arthrotomy is performed 3–4 mm medial to the patellar tendon. The incision must be large enough for adequate positioning of a stifle distractor; with experience, good results can generally be obtained via smaller arthrotomies (mini-arthrotomy).

Following stifle arthrotomy, a stifle distractor is positioned between the femoral intercondylar fossa and the cranial aspect of the tibial plateau to provide optimal exposure of the joint and cranial subluxation of the tibia. The visibility of intra-articular structures may be improved by partial excision of the infrapatellar fat pad or by the use of Senn retractors over the infrapatellar fat pad.

A blunt probe is used to palpate the entire surface of the medial and lateral menisci and the tip is then hooked under the caudal pole of each meniscus abaxial to the meniscotibial ligament and pulled cranially to assess integrity. The probe is used to evaluate the integrity of the caudal cruciate ligament. Any signs of cartilage disease on the femoral condyles, meniscal injury and or changes in the caudal cruciate ligament should be recorded.

Where SMI is suspected in a patient with an almost intact CrCL at the time of surgery, transection of the CrCL remnants is strongly recommended; this facilitates visualisation and palpation of the medial and lateral menisci and potentially treats cases with chronic pain associated with progressive degeneration of the CrCL despite previous surgical intervention for dynamic stabilisation of the stifle. In the author's experience, Boxers seem to be overrepresented in this group of dogs with chronic stifle pain after TPLO surgery in which cruciate ligament remnants have been left in situ. Therefore, complete excision at the time of first surgery is recommended.

MEDIAL MENISCAL RELEASE

Meniscal release (MR) allows the caudal horn of the medial meniscus to displace caudally, avoiding impingement between the medial femoral condyle and the tibial condyle, thereby eliminating its wedge effect. Although TPLO results in changes in pressure distribution to the caudal compartment and may reduce the space for the meniscus during extreme flexion of the joint, postoperative meniscal injuries are more likely to be caused by persistent instability (rotational or translational) or misdiagnosis at the time of the first surgery (latent tear) (Kim et al., 2009).

Two forms of MR are described in the literature: meniscotibial ligament meniscotomy or axial release; and mid-body or abaxial release, with the meniscotomy located just caudal to the medial collateral ligament and the incision angled at the tubercle of Gerdi. No significant difference was found between the intrameniscal area (IMA) of abaxial compared with axial meniscal release in a cadaveric study (Kennedy et al., 2005). It is the author's preference to perform an axial release, as subjectively, direct visualisation of the caudal meniscotibial ligament is superior, meaning that the transection is better controlled and thus safer than during abaxial release.

Axial release

A meniscal probe is used to apply cranial traction to the ligament to facilitate its safe transection. Care is taken to identify the caudal cruciate ligament and to hook the caudal meniscotibial ligament to avoid iatrogenic damage to the caudal cruciate ligament. A Beaver blade is preferably used to cut the meniscotibial ligament from caudal to cranial onto the meniscal probe (Fig. 7). Confirmation of complete meniscal release must be ascertained by palpation of the free edge with the use of a meniscal probe. Alternatively, a meniscal hook knife can be used for transection of the ligament.

Abaxial (mid-body) release

A number 11 scalpel blade is preferably used to cut the meniscus immediately caudal to the medial collateral ligament, aiming for the tubercle of Gerdi on the proximolateral aspect of the tibia (Fig. 7). Similarly, the use of a meniscal probe to evaluate complete release is mandatory.

Systematic meniscal release is not recommended routinely and it is the author's preference to perform a release in patients presented for SMI when meniscal inspection does not reveal a clear meniscal injury and the CrCL has been fully excised.

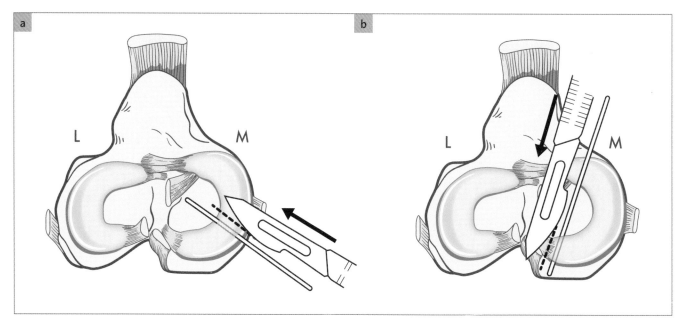

Figure 7. Diagram illustrating abaxial meniscal release (note the scalpel blade is introduced in the joint caudal to the medial collateral ligament and with 45 degrees of cranial angulation) (a) and axial release (note the meniscal probe hooked under the caudal meniscotibial ligament and on a second step the scalpel blade cutting on the meniscal probe) (b). Adapted from: Tobias KM, Johnston SA, *Veterinary Surgery: Small Animal*, 2nd ed. (2017).

MENISCAL SURGERY

Preservation of meniscal function is key. Abnormal tissues should be excised, while preserving as much intact meniscus as possible (Fig. 8).

Partial meniscectomy

Partial meniscectomy is generally recommended for meniscal tears that do not extend to the rim. Removal of the damaged free or axial section is performed, while preserving the ligamentous attachments of the meniscus. Ideal meniscal injuries for this treatment are vertical longitudinal tears, "bucket handle" and flap tears.

A pair of mosquito artery forceps or a meniscal probe can be used to grab or apply tension to the axial/free portion of the meniscus. A Beaver blade or a number 11 scalpel blade can be used to transect the most cranial and caudal part of the free portion of the meniscus. Inspection is performed with a meniscal probe as it is not unusual to find a second or subsequent longitudinal tears in some patients. The joint is flushed and closed as per routine.

Caudal hemimeniscectomy

This procedure involves excision of the caudal pole of the medial meniscus. This is generally used for complex tears,

degenerative tears and radial tears. The caudal meniscotibial ligament is carefully transected as explained earlier (see *Meniscal inspection*, p. 74), taking care to protect the caudal cruciate ligament. The caudal pole of the meniscus is then grasped with a pair of artery forceps and its most axial part is cut where it overlies the tibial plateau. The procedure is finished by transverse excision of the caudal pole of the medial meniscus as cranial as is necessary to remove all pathological meniscal tissue. The joint is flushed and closed as per routine.

Total meniscectomy

Total meniscectomy involves excision of the whole medial or lateral meniscus by releasing it from its cranial, caudal and abaxial ligaments. This is an unusual procedure that should be reserved for cases with longitudinal tears involving the cranial and caudal horns of a meniscus, or that have suffered multiple ligamentous injuries in the stifle resulting in the meniscus becoming unstable. The caudal meniscus is excised as described for caudal hemimeniscectomy; the cranial meniscotibial ligament is then excised as well. Abaxial excision of all abnormal meniscal tissues along the cranial and caudal pole of the affected meniscus is performed. The joint is flushed and closed as per routine.

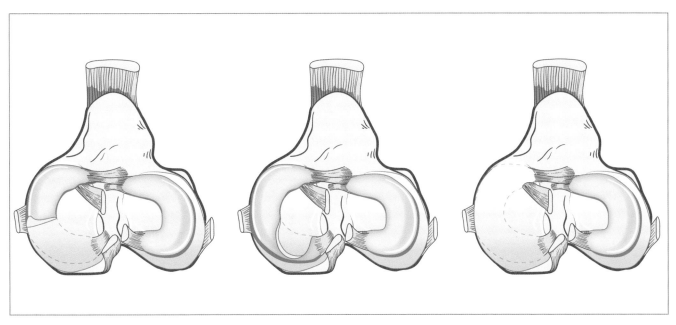

Figure 8. Proximodistal view of a right tibial plateau following partial, caudal or medial meniscectomy. Adapted from: Tobias KM, Johnston SA, *Veterinary Surgery: Small Animal*, 2nd ed. (2017).

POSTOPERATIVE MANAGEMENT

Perioperative antibiotic therapy is given to all patients and discontinued at the end of the surgical procedure. Oral nonsteroidal anti-inflammatory drugs (NSAIDs) are provided for a minimum of 14 days. The limb is not usually bandaged and it is recommended that cryotherapy is applied every 4–6 hours after surgery for the first 72 hours.

Strict rest is prescribed for 6 weeks (by confinement in a big cage or small room) with no jumping, running, walking on slippery surfaces, off-lead exercise, steps or stairs allowed. The patient can go outside on the lead for 10 minutes 3–4 times a day for toilet purposes for the first 2 weeks. The skin sutures or staples are removed after 10–14 days. Provided good clinical progression is seen, lead exercise can be increased by 5 minutes per walk each week for 4 weeks, followed by slow reintroduction of off-lead exercise over an additional 4-week period. Physiotherapy and regular hydrotherapy is strongly recommended for these patients.

OUTCOME

The time taken for clinical signs to improve or resolve is variable; in the author's experience, dogs with SMI and partial meniscectomy require a minimum of 12 weeks.

Overall, the current literature offers contradictory information regarding long-term outcomes after meniscal surgery. Several studies have reported resolution or improvement in lameness after partial meniscectomy for treatment of SMI (Stein and Schmoekel, 2008; Dymond, 2010; Gatineau et al., 2011; Kalff, 2011); however, it is well known that meniscectomy precipitates osteoarthritis and it has been suggested that its severity is associated with the degree of meniscal excision (Cox and Cordell, 1977; Franklin et al., 2010; Pozzi et al., 2010).

Some studies have shown similar outcomes in dogs undergoing a partial meniscectomy compared with those in which the meniscus was intact at the time of stifle surgery (Thieman et al., 2006; Stein and Schmoekel, 2008). Moreover, no significant difference was reported in the severity of postoperative radiographic osteoarthritis between dogs that underwent meniscectomy and dogs with intact menisci in three studies (Rayward et al., 2004; Ertelt and Fehr 2009; Morgan et al., 2010), and there was no significant difference in force plate analysis between dogs undergoing partial meniscectomy and those with intact menisci at the time of surgery (Johnson, 2004; Voss, 2008; Morgan et al., 2010).

These results are in contradiction with other reports based on owner questionnaires, where dogs with intact menisci at the time of surgery had better outcomes when compared to those that underwent a partial meniscectomy (Smith and Torg, 1985; Innes et al., 2000; Gatineau et al., 2011). Another study showed a smaller proportion of dogs with partial meniscectomy and concurrent cruciate ligament disease surgery achieving similar results to clinically normal dogs during force plate analysis (Conzemius et al., 2005).

COMPLICATIONS

Complications associated with meniscal surgery may be seen as for any case undergoing arthrotomy (surgical site infection, septic arthritis, wound breakdown, seroma, etc.) in addition to long-term lameness.

03

THE TARSUS

INTRODUCTION

The need for surgery in the tarsal joint is relatively uncommon in companion dogs and cats. The most common indications for surgery are related to trauma or pathology of the supporting tendinous or ligamentous structures.

> Some of the most common surgical conditions affecting the tarsal joint include traumatic luxations and fractures, degenerative plantar ligament conditions, osteochondrosis and pathology of the common calcaneal (Achilles) tendon mechanism.

It is important to have a detailed understanding of the complex anatomy of the tarsus before performing surgery on this joint. Briefly, the tarsal joint is made of seven individual bones: the calcaneus, talus, central tarsal bone and four numbered tarsal bones. The tarsal bones are arranged in three irregular rows, with the calcaneus and talus forming the proximal row. The six main articulations of the tarsus are the talocrural, talocalcaneal, talocalcaneocentral, calcaneoquartal, centrodistal and tarsometatarsal joints (Fig. 1). The talocalcaneocentral and calcaneoquartal joints form the proximal intertarsal joint. About 90 % of the range of motion of the joint in the sagittal plane occurs at the level of the talocrural joint; motion in the other tarsal joints is minimal.

The joint is stabilised by a very extensive ligamentous and thick fascial support structure. This includes individual ligaments connecting all tarsal bones, dorsal and plantar thickening of the fibrous joint capsule, and medial and lateral collateral ligaments. The malleoli also contribute to the stability of the joint.

The medial and lateral tarsal collateral ligaments in the dog each consist of three individual components. The medial collateral ligament complex has a long component that spans superficially from the medial malleolus to the central tarsal and first tarsal bones, a short tibiocentral component and a short thick tibiotalar component that runs across the other two. Assessment of medial collateral stability during orthopaedic examination must be carried out with the tarsus in flexion and extension, since the first two components are taut in extension and the short tibiotalar ligament is taut

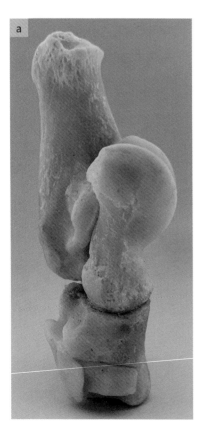
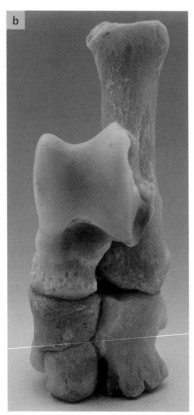
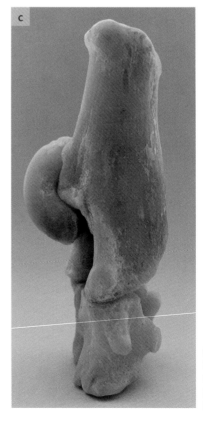

Figure 1. Medial (a), dorsal (b) and (c) views of the tarsal bones.

The author of this chapter would like to acknowledge his colleagues Elena Addison and Esteve González and his coauthors for their help at various stages of the writing of this chapter.

in flexion. The lateral collateral ligament complex also has a long component that spans superficially from the lateral malleolus to the fourth tarsal bone and the base of the fifth metatarsal bone, a short calcaneofibular component and a short talofibular component; the first two of these are taut in extension and the talofibular component is taut in flexion (Aron and Purinton, 1985a). Cats lack the long component of both medial and lateral ligaments, having only the straight and oblique components (Montavon et al., 2009).

The angle of the normal tarsocrural joint (Fig. 2) during weight-bearing is reported to be 135–145 degrees in dogs and 115–125 degrees in cats (DeCamp et al., 2015). The normal range of motion has been reported to be 39 degrees in flexion to 164 degrees in extension in the normal canine joint (Jaegger and Marcellin-Little, 2002), and 22 degrees in flexion to 167 degrees in extension in the normal feline joint (Jaeger et al., 2007).

Tarsal joint function is intrinsically related to the mechanism of the common calcaneal tendon (Fig. 3), which comprises the superficial digital flexor tendon (SDFT), the gastrocnemius tendon and the combined tendon of the gracilis, semitendinosus, and biceps muscles. The SDFT runs superficially and widens as it nears the calcaneus, where it attaches, before continuing distally to insert on the plantar aspects of the phalanges. The tendon of the gastrocnemius, which constitutes the main component, has two muscular heads that combine into a single tendon before inserting on to the dorsal surface of the calcaneus. The combined tendon of the gracilis, semitendinosus, and biceps muscles inserts onto the calcaneus mainly as part of the crural fascia.

The arterial blood supply to the tarsus is from the cranial tibial artery and the plantar branches of the saphenous artery. The cranial tibial artery continues as the dorsal pedal artery at the level of the talocrural joint before giving rise to the dorsal metatarsal arteries distally. A large perforating branch arises from the dorsal metatarsal artery II, which courses between the proximal aspect of the second and third metatarsal bones in a dorsal to plantar direction, and anastomoses with the lateral plantar branch of the saphenous artery. The resulting vessel will give rise to the plantar metatarsal arteries, the main blood supply to the paw distal to the tarsus. Branches of both the tibial (plantar) and common peroneal (dorsal) nerves provide motor innervation to the joint.

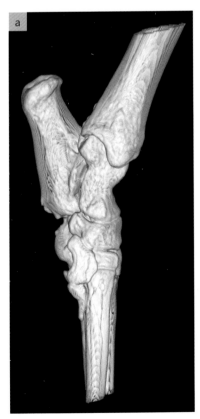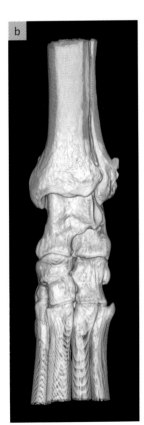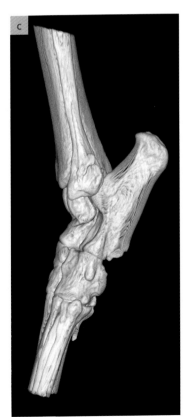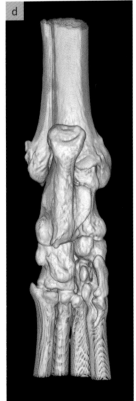

Figure 2. Three-dimensional computed tomography (CT) reconstruction images of the distal tibia, tarsal joint and proximal metatarsal bones illustrating the relationship between various bones and joints. Medial (a), dorsal (b), lateral (c) and plantar (d) views are seen.

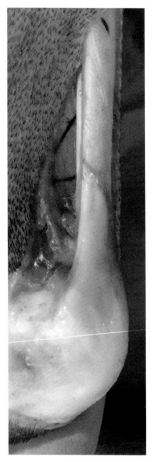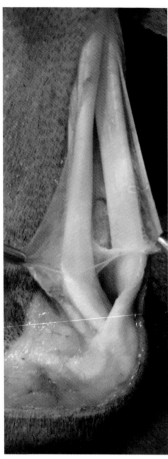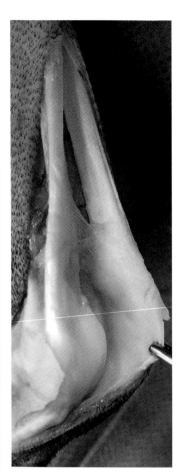

Figure 3. Dissected specimen of the insertion area of the common calcaneal tendon in a medium-sized dog with progressive elevation of the superficial digital flexor tendon from the tendon of insertion of the gastrocnemius muscle.

Orthopaedic examination of the tarsal joint is carried out in a standard fashion. The joints are palpated for pain, bone or soft tissue swelling, crepitus, heat and effusion. Joint range of motion is assessed and the joints are manipulated for evidence of dorsal, plantar or mediolateral instability. The contralateral limb should be assessed for comparison. Many conditions affecting the tarsal joint are bilateral with different degrees of clinical effect. The common calcaneal tendons are carefully palpated, particularly at the level of their insertion. Diagnostic investigation of tarsal pathology often includes orthogonal radiographic imaging of the affected or both tarsal joints. Computed tomography may be required to identify elusive

fractures and stressed radiographic views are useful to identify the level of instability in cases of ligamentous injury. Joint arthrocentesis is indicated when inflammatory or infectious conditions are possible differential diagnoses. Ultrasound examination allows further assessment of common calcaneal tendon injuries.

The four main surgical approaches to the tarsal joint are lateral, medial (with or without medial malleolar osteotomy), plantar and dorsomedial (Johnson et al., 2005; Montavon et al., 2009; Johnson, 2013). A more detailed description of the intricate anatomy, functional characteristics and various surgical approaches to the tarsal joint can be found elsewhere (Miller et al., 2013; Tobias et al., 2013).

COMMON CALCANEAL TENDON MECHANISM AND INJURY REPAIR

INTRODUCTION

The two most common presentations of common calcaneal tendon injury are acute traumatic rupture and chronic degenerative injury. Chronic degenerative injuries tend to exclusively affect the tendon of the gastrocnemius, while the SDFT is frequently also affected in acute traumatic injuries. The tendon components involved, the location and severity of the injury and the time elapsed since it occurred should all be taken into account when planning treatment and to inform prognosis (Meutstege, 1993) (Box 1).

Acute injuries typically occur following direct trauma to some part of the musculotendinous unit or impact injury causing tendon avulsion from the calcaneus. They can cause various degrees of lameness and tarsal hyperflexion (plantigrade stance) on weight-bearing. Diagnosis is usually made by palpation of the tendon and ultrasound examination. A wound may be present. Complete transection or rupture of the common calcaneal tendon requires surgical repair.

The chronic form of common calcaneal tendon injury usually occurs by avulsion of the tendon of insertion of the gastrocnemius muscle from the tuber calcanei (type IIc lesions). It tends to affect medium- and large-breed dogs and causes progressive lameness and plantigrade stance in the affected limb. It is often bilateral and usually there is no history of trauma. The digits are often kept in a flexed position (in a characteristic "clawing" position) due to preservation and stretching of the tendon of the superficial digital flexor muscle during plantigrade stance. Nonpainful thickening of the area of insertion of the common calcaneal tendon is usually present and the diagnosis can be confirmed by ultrasound. Radiographs can often confirm the presence of focal swelling of the distal tendon and enthesiophytes in the area of insertion onto the calcaneus. The cause of this condition is poorly understood but chronic low-grade trauma is suspected. Management of the chronic form will depend on the severity of the condition (Swaim et al., 2015).

Common calcaneal tendon pathology in cats is uncommon but management is similar to that in dogs. It is important to consider diabetic neuromyopathy and neurological lesions

> **Box 1. Classification of common calcaneal tendon injuries.**
>
> Tendon components involved
> - Gastrocnemius tendon
> - SDFT*
>
> Chronicity of the injury
> - Acute: within 48 hours
> - Subacute: between 2 and 21 days
> - Chronic: more than 21 days
>
> Location and severity of the injury:
> - Type I: complete tendon rupture
> - Type II: subdivided into three subtypes
>   - Type IIa: musculotendinous rupture
>   - Type IIb: common calcaneal tendon rupture with paratenon preservation
>   - Type IIc: partial gastrocnemius tendon avulsion with intact SDFT
> - Type III: tendinosis and peritendinitis
>
> *SDFT: superficial digital flexor tendon

as differential diagnoses for a plantigrade stance in this species. In a recent report of 21 feline cases, only half had a history of trauma while two-thirds had tendinosseous avulsions (Cervi et al., 2010).

INDICATIONS FOR SURGERY

Patients with evidence of acute complete tendon rupture or increased tarsal flexion should be considered surgical candidates.

Optimal management of tears of the musculotendinous junction or muscle belly of the gastrocnemius will depend on the time elapsed since the injury occurred and its severity. Surgical repair should be attempted for those acute and traumatic tears that cause plantigrade stance.

More chronic injuries can also be repaired, although arthrodesis may be a more definitive treatment option, particularly in degenerative ruptures as well as those in which previous attempts at repair have failed.

Chronic tendinitis, core lesions or incomplete tears can be treated conservatively, although many of these cases will eventually require pantarsal arthrodesis. A case of successful treatment of gastrocnemius tendon strain using autologous mesenchymal stem cells and a custom orthosis has been reported (Case et al., 2013).

SURGICAL PLANNING

Following acute injury, primary repair of each individual transected component of the musculotendinous unit, in conjunction with temporary immobilisation of the tibiotarsal joint, is advised. Temporary immobilisation can be achieved using a transarticular external skeletal fixator (ESF), a calcaneotibial screw, or a cast/splint with the hock in extension. Radiographs that include the entire length of the tibia and metatarsal bones are required if placement of a transarticular ESF is anticipated (see *Transarticular external skeletal fixation in the tarsal joint,* p. 97).

Primary repair and temporary immobilisation of the joint is also advised for most chronic injuries of the common calcaneal tendon, and the same preoperative planning applies (Fig. 1); however, chronic tissue fibrosis and gastrocnemius muscle contracture may prevent the necessary contact of the tendon with the calcaneus without excessive tension, and lengthening and augmentation techniques may be required. The use of these techniques must be planned before surgery. Described techniques include V–Y plasty and use of fascial grafts (i.e. fascia lata) (Sivacolundhu et al., 2001), use of autogenous muscles or tendons (i.e. semitendinosus muscle or peroneal tendons) (Baltzer and Rist, 2009; Diserens and Venzin, 2015) or use of artificial implants (i.e. bone plates or polypropylene meshes) (Swiderski et al., 2005). Use of a polyethylene terephthalate implant for management of large gaps due to gastrocnemius contraction or loss of substance has also recently been reported (Morton et al., 2015).

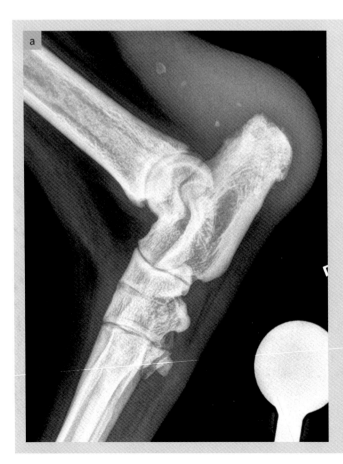
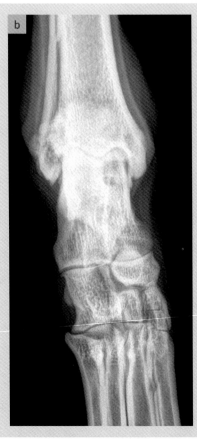

Figure 1. Preoperative mediolateral (a) and dorsoplantar (b) radiographs of the right tarsal joint of a 6-year-old Pointer affected with degenerative injury of the common calcaneal tendon. Marked soft tissue swelling and multiple areas of dystrophic mineralisation at the insertional area of the gastrocnemius tendon are seen. The calcaneus is irregular proximally and enthesiophytes are also present.

SURGICAL TECHNIQUES

CHRONIC COMMON CALCANEAL TENDON MECHANISM INJURY

Key to tendon repair are gentle tissue handling and creation of an environment conducive to healing, with progressive loading of the tendon over time.

The entire limb is clipped and aseptically prepared, including the foot, which is covered with a foot bandage. For unilateral procedures the patient is placed in lateral recumbency with a hanging limb technique. A second sterile foot bandage is placed at the time of draping.

A standard lateral approach to the calcaneus is performed (Johnson, 2013). A curved skin incision is made from the distal quarter of the tibia distally, passing lateral to the plantar midline until it reaches the distal calcaneus. Following dissection of the subcutaneous tissue, the deep crural fascia and lateral retinacular attachment of the SDFT are sharply incised between the SDFT and the gastrocnemius tendon. The incision of the tendon sheath can now be extended proximally and distally as required to allow for medial retraction of the SDFT and exposure of the distal gastrocnemius tendon and the proximal calcaneus (Figs. 2 and 3).

It is important to minimise any excessive traction and trauma to the gastrocnemius tendon. Approximation to the distal end of the calcaneus is aided by extension of the tarsal joint and flexion of the stifle. Any traction to the tendon is done with the help of needles or Kirschner wires used as skewers, inserted 5–10 mm away from the distal end of the tendon. The tendon end is now assessed and any fibrous (scar) tissue is excised to allow for direct tendon-to-bone apposition. This may require conservative sharp transection of the tip of the tendon (fibrous cap of tissue). Presence of abundant fibrous tissue and adhesions is common in chronic cases and makes

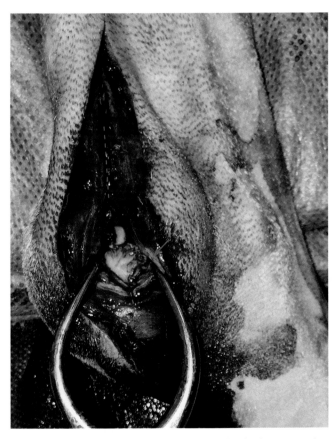

Figure 2. Patient from Figure 1. Lateral approach to the distal common calcaneal tendon and proximal calcaneus. The deep fascia has been sharply incised near the point of insertion of the tendon (arrow) and the incision can now be extended proximally and distally (dotted lines) to allow medial retraction of the superficial digital flexor tendon (SDFT) and deep fascia (star). Near complete avulsion of the gastrocnemius component of the common calcaneal tendon can be observed. The SDFT is intact.

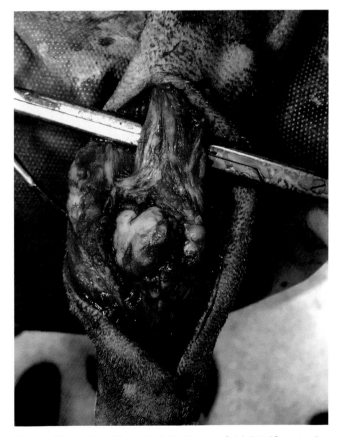

Figure 3. Plantar view of the surgical site. The superficial digital flexor tendon (SDFT) has been retracted medially (star), improving the visualisation of the tendon of the gastrocnemius, which can be seen almost completely detached from the tuber calcanei. Note the marked thickening around the SDFT and presence of a fibrous tissue cap at the distal end of the tendon of the gastrocnemius secondary to chronic inflammation.

the identification of the different components of the tendon difficult. A small transverse bone tunnel can now be drilled in a lateromedial direction 3–4 mm distal to the proximal end of the calcaneus using a 1.5 mm drill bit. This tunnel will be used to anchor the gastrocnemius tendon to the calcaneus. Point-to-point bone-holding forceps can also be used from the calcaneus to the cranial tibia to keep the talocrural joint extended. If placement of a positional calcaneotibial screw is planned (this is not a lag screw), a second bone tunnel is now drilled in a plantarodorsal direction from the caudal cortex of the proximal calcaneus and through the tibia proximal to the talocrural joint (Fig. 4). Slight lateromedial angulation is necessary to penetrate the centre of the caudal cortex of the tibia. The use of a washer will prevent the head of the screw form sinking into the calcaneus. For medium and large-breed dogs, 3.5 and 4.5 mm screws are commonly used; 2 mm screws are used for cats. Alternatively, use of a transarticular ESF, cast or splinted bandage may be considered for temporary stabilisation of the tendon repair.

The debrided gastrocnemius tendon is now repaired with a modification of the three-loop pulley technique (Moores et al., 2004a) (Box 2). Long-term absorbable monofilament suture material such as polydioxanone can be used.

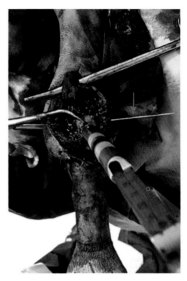

Figure 4. Plantar view of the surgical site. Two bone tunnels have been created in the calcaneus. A small Kirschner wire has been placed through the transverse tunnel that will be used for reattachment of the gastrocnemius tendon to the calcaneus (arrow). Following talocrural joint immobilisation in extension with point-to-point bone holding forceps (star), a calcaneotibial bone tunnel has been drilled and the length of the positional screw needed is being measured with a depth gauge.

The recommended size of polydioxanone is 0 USP in large dogs and 2-0 in small dogs and cats, tied with a surgeon's throw followed by three square knots. It is important to achieve good apposition of the two ends since gap formation over 3 mm can significantly delay tendon healing and increase the risk of failure of the repair in the first 6 weeks following surgery (Moores et al., 2004b).

Box. 2. Modified three-loop pulley pattern technique.

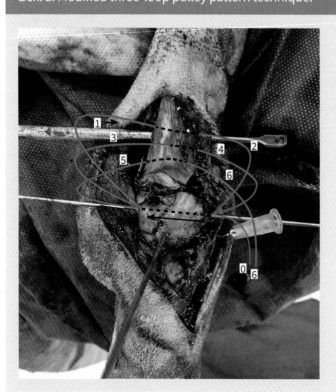

The following sequence is followed for placement of the modified three-loop pulley suture.

0 to 1: The suture is passed in a lateral-to-medial direction through the bone tunnel.

1 to 2: Medial-to-lateral "far" bite through the tendon.

2 to 3: Lateral-to-medial pass through the bone tunnel.

3 to 4: Caudomedial-to-craniolateral "middle" bite through the tendon, at approximately 60 degrees (anticlockwise) from the first bite.

4 to 5: Lateral-to-medial pass through the bone tunnel.

5 to 6: Craniomedial-to-caudolateral "near" bite through the tendon, at approximately 60 degrees (clockwise) from the first bite.

0 and 6: The suture ends are tied together.

Figure 5. Same patient as in Figures 1–4. Plantar view of the surgical site. Note that if a calcaneotibial screw and washer are used, they should be secured before placement of the anchor suture. The distal end of the gastrocnemius tendon has already been debrided of fibrous tissue.

The joint is now lavaged and the surgical wound is closed. It is important to ensure a secure closure to the deep fascial and retinacular incision to prevent medial luxation of the SDFT. Subcutaneous and skin layers are closed routinely.

ACUTE INJURIES OF THE COMMON CALCANEAL TENDON MECHANISM

Acute injuries are managed similarly, although both the gastrocnemius tendon and the SDFT are usually transected and are repaired separately. First the gastrocnemius tendon is repaired with a standard three-loop pulley technique (tendon-to-tendon repair). Apposition of the tendon ends can be improved by placement of several horizontal mattress sutures of a smaller gauge absorbable suture material (i.e. 2-0 or 3-0 USP) around the circumference of the repair. The SDFT is repaired next. Being a flat tendon, the use of a locking loop suture pattern is more appropriate. It is important to remember that, for the suture to tighten on the fibre bundles, the transverse component must be superficial to the longitudinal one (Tomlinson and Moore, 1982). The rest of the procedure is similar to that described for the chronic form of common calcaneal tendon injury.

POSTOPERATIVE MANAGEMENT

Postoperative radiographs are taken if any radiopaque implants have been placed (Fig. 6).

Standard cold packing of the surgical wound every 4 hours for the first 3 days postoperatively and use of non-steroidal anti-inflammatory drugs (NSAIDs) for the first 2 weeks are advised. The calcaneotibial screw or transarticular ESF can be removed after 3 weeks and a splinted bandage is applied for another 3 weeks. This is followed by application of a soft padded bandage for 3 weeks, and 3 months of restricted exercise and physical rehabilitation therapy. Bandages must be checked daily by the owner and changed weekly by a veterinary surgeon. Alternatively, the calcaneotibial screw can remain in place for 6–8 weeks, or a cast or splinted bandage can be used for the first 7 weeks. No method has been proven superior to others and it is a matter of the surgeon's preference. However, complete joint immobilisation and rest of the injured tendon for more than 3–4 weeks is counterproductive and leads to muscle atrophy, chondromalacia and joint ankylosis. Cage or room rest and controlled lead exercise for the first 6 months is also advised.

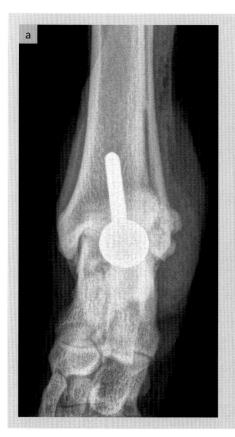
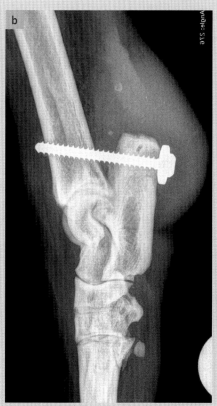

Figure 6. Postoperative mediolateral (a) and dorsoplantar (b) radiographs of the same patient following common calcaneal tendon repair and calcaneotibial screw placement, showing correct placement of a 4.5 mm positional cortical screw and a washer. The very proximal transverse calcaneal bone tunnel used for anchoring of the gastrocnemius tendon can also be seen in both views.

Management is similar for cats, with 3 weeks of complete immobilisation, followed by application of a splinted bandage for another 3 weeks and a final 6–10 weeks of house confinement.

OUTCOME

The outcome following repair of common calcaneal tendon lesions is reported to be good to excellent in 72–94 % of canine patients. Dogs with injuries of less than 21 days' duration may have a better functional outcome (Nielsen and Pluhar, 2006; Corr et al., 2010). In a study in dogs that compared the use of a transarticular ESF with that of a splint or cast after primary repair (with or without placement of a calcaneotibial screw), no statistical differences were identified in the overall complication rate, duration of immobilisation or functional outcome (Nielsen and Pluhar, 2006).

In cats, traumatic and atraumatic types of injury were equally represented in a retrospective study and the overall outcome following surgery was similar, with a long-term success of 84 % (Cervi et al., 2010).

COMPLICATIONS

A retrospective study comparing postoperative tibiotarsal immobilisation methods following common calcaneal tendon repair in 28 dogs reported that most complications were associated with tibiotarsal stabilisation, not with the primary repair of the tendon, with an overall complication rate of 46 % (Nielsen and Pluhar, 2006). All major complications were reported in the group immobilised with a transarticular ESF (31 % of major complication rate) and included osteomyelitis and pin loosening, bone fractures and breakage of pins or acrylic fixator bars. Minor complications in the study included superficial pin tract infections, skin impingement against ESF clamps, bandage-induced dermatitis or wounds, and splint breakage.

In another retrospective study comparing 45 dogs managed with primary repair protected mostly with a calcaneotibial screw and a cast, only 8 % of screws had to be replaced due to bending or breakage (Corr et al., 2010). Overall complication rate was 35 %, with a third of those being major complications. Common complications included skin infections and pressure wounds.

Complications in cats were reported in around 33 % of cases and were also found to be related to the method of tibiotarsal stabilisation, and almost invariably associated with the use of an ESF (Cervi et al., 2010). The authors of the study recommended the use of external coaptation as the optimal method of immobilisation in this species, although calcaneotibial screws were not used in this study.

LUXATIONS OF THE TARSAL JOINT

Stability of the tarsal joint relies on the presence of very extensive ligamentous and fascial support. The tarsal collateral ligaments provide much of the mediolateral joint stability, and a detailed description of their anatomy can be found in the introduction of this chapter. The fibrous component of the joint capsule spans from the distal tibia to the proximal aspect of the metatarsal bones and contains the tarsal ligaments. This thickened fibrous fascia is particularly well developed on the plantar aspect, and accounts for most of the plantar stability of the intertarsal and tarsometatarsal joints. The tarsus is more than three times longer than the carpus and sustains tremendous propulsive forces, making it susceptible to stress injuries. Furthermore, the paucity of soft tissue protection makes it susceptible to fractures and shearing injuries following trauma.

> Tarsal joint instability can be caused by loss of integrity of one or more supporting structures, including collateral ligaments, plantar and dorsal ligaments, and malleoli.

Tibiotarsal joint instability is typically caused by trauma, including shearing injuries and closed dislocations secondary to malleolar fracture and/or collateral ligamentous injury. It results in mediolateral joint instability due to loss of collateral ligamentous support. Concurrent injuries secondary to trauma are common and a systematic and multisystem approach to the diagnosis and management of these cases is required.

Intertarsal and tarsometatarsal subluxations and luxations typically cause joint hyperflexion (plantigrade stance) secondary to loss of plantar ligamentous support. However, they differ in that, while tarsometatarsal pathology is usually traumatic, most intertarsal pathology is suspected to be degenerative or secondary to chronic stress injury.

Conservative management of second- and third-degree ligamentous injuries with rest, with or without external coaptation, is usually associated with a poor outcome, and surgery is advised (DeCamp et al., 2015). Second- and third-degree ligament injuries involve a partial or complete tear of the affected ligament, respectively, and cause joint instability.

Careful manipulation of the affected joint may help confirm the presence and direction of the luxation (hyperflexion, hyperextension, varus or valgus deviation). Orthogonal radiographs may identify concurrent fractures. Stressed radiographic views may also be required for subtle subluxations and to help determine the anatomical structures involved and direction of the luxation.

TYPES OF LUXATIONS

TIBIOTARSAL SUBLUXATION AND LUXATION
Traumatic tibiotarsal joint instability can occur secondary to shearing injury, or to closed malleolar and/or collateral ligament injury. Shearing injuries are most common and can result in various degrees of damage to the malleoli, collateral ligaments, joint capsule and bony support.

Treatment options for the management of talocrural instability include external coaptation, primary ligamentous repair, prosthetic ligamentous reconstruction, use of a transarticular ESF, arthrodesis and amputation. The choice of treatment will depend on the patient (i.e. weight and character) and the type and severity of tissue damage.

Closed traumatic collateral ligament injuries and malleolar fractures
Closed luxations can be caused by fracture of the malleolus (Fig. 1) or ligament failure. Any combination of the two can occur within the same joint with bilateral injuries (i.e. affecting the medial and lateral aspect of the same joint). Malleolar fractures heal more readily and are associated with a better prognosis than collateral ligament ruptures (Tobias and Johnston, 2013).

Malleolar fractures are considered articular fractures and early repair with internal rigid fixation is mandatory. The repair is protected postoperatively with application of a splinted bandage or transarticular ESF for 2–4 weeks. Collateral ligamentous ruptures can be treated by prosthetic ligamentous reconstruction, with or without primary repair, followed by application of a splinted bandage or transarticular ESF for 4–6 weeks. Primary repair should be attempted if there is enough remaining tissue, although this is uncommon.

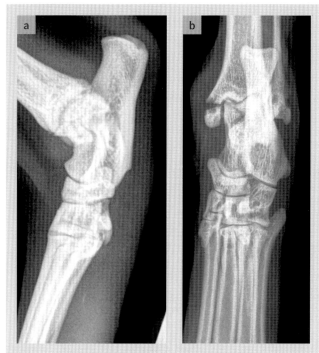

Figure 1. Mediolateral (a) and dorsoplantar (b) radiographs of a closed medial malleolar fracture in a 4-year-old domestic shorthair cat following trauma. Note the presence of soft tissue swelling around the fracture site.

Prosthetic reconstruction has been associated with major complications (mostly implant infection and failure) and owners should be made aware of this prior to surgery (Diamond et al., 1999; Beever et al., 2016). Failed prosthetic reconstruction may require implant replacement, or implant removal and joint arthrodesis, if instability remains. The techniques for primary ligamentous repair or prosthetic reconstruction of the tarsal collateral ligaments are not described in this chapter, although this information can be found elsewhere (Aron and Purinton, 1985b; Montavon et al., 2009; Swaim et al., 2015).

In feline patients, good outcomes have been reported for isolated injuries of a single collateral ligament following repair or prosthetic replacement. Outcome for bilateral (in the same joint) and shearing injuries is less consistent due to the greater magnitude of trauma, which results in increased joint damage and frequent presence of concurrent injuries (Schmökel et al., 1994; Montavon et al., 2009).

Shearing injury

Degloving and shearing injuries are frequently the result of the patient being dragged by a moving vehicle and often involve the distal limbs. The medial aspect of the tarsal and metatarsal areas is most commonly affected. Shearing of deep tissues occurs with greater trauma and includes skin, tendons and ligament, joint capsule, bone and neurovascular structures. About 75 % of all shearing injuries result in bone or joint exposure and slightly more than half have joint instability (Beardsley and Schrader, 1995). Furthermore, bacteria and debris are often embedded in the remaining tissue, which is also compromised due to crushing and trauma.

A complete description of the management of the soft tissue and orthopaedic aspects of these injuries is beyond the scope of this book. However, some guidelines are given below. The following must be determined for any shearing wound within the first 2–4 days following trauma:

- Life-threatening injuries. These must be identified and treated on admission and may require a delay in the management of any wounds. Wounds should be protected with a sterile bandage until the patient's condition is stable.
- Degree of vascular and neurological damage. Surprisingly few cases have severe vascular compromise to the distal limb or neurological deficits. Blood supply to the distal limb can be confirmed with the use of Doppler ultrasound. Severe neurological deficits may require limb amputation, lifelong use of an orthosis, or joint arthrodesis.
- Integrity of the periarticular support structures and degree of joint instability.
- Extent of bone loss and loss of articular cartilage.
- Extent of skin loss. The full extent may not be apparent at the time of initial presentation and daily assessment is often required for the first 2–4 days.

Thorough wound examination under heavy sedation or general anaesthesia is performed as soon as is deemed safe for the patient. Orthogonal and stressed radiographs are taken as required at this time. Initial wide hair clipping, removal of foreign debris, conservative surgical debridement of devitalised tissue and thorough wound lavage is followed by appropriate sterile wound coverage. Unstable joints may require splinting or early placement of a transarticular ESF. The use of a broad-spectrum bactericidal antibiotic is indicated until bacteriology results are available, until presence of healthy granulation tissue, or until surgical closure of the wound. A bacteriology swab sample can be taken following initial wound lavage.

Repeated wound lavage, strategic tissue debridement and open wound management with wet-to-dry dressings or advanced wound dressings such as alginate, film, foam, hydrocolloid or hydrogel dressings is repeated daily until there is presence of healthy granulation tissue or the wound can be closed (i.e. a clean wound with healthy tissue and no evidence of infection). The optimal timing for definitive management of bony injuries is determined by the extent of the soft tissue injuries. With severe injuries this usually takes 3–5 days of open wound management (Diamond et al., 1999), although it may take longer.

Treatment options for definitive closure of the skin defect include primary wound closure, second intention healing and use of skin grafts. Although small wounds can be sutured closed or allowed to heal by second intention, most large wounds will need skin grafting. Allowing wounds to heal by contraction and epithelisation result in thin and friable epithelial coverage that may compromise range of motion, particularly when wounds extend to the flexion surface of the joint. Negative pressure wound therapy can be used to promote granulation tissue formation, or following skin grafting (Box 1).

The choice of technique for definitive joint stabilisation depends on the type and severity of the injury. It has been stated that joint salvage can be attempted if over 50 % of the joint surface is viable (Tobias and Johnston, 2013). Collateral reconstruction (malleolar or ligamentous) and temporary joint stabilisation can be considered in mild cases. However, prosthetic ligamentous reconstruction, particularly when used as part of the management of open injuries, is significantly associated with severe long-term complications and its use

has been questioned. There is evidence suggesting that the short and long-term outcome following surgical stabilisation of tarsocrural instability with a temporary transarticular ESF alone is similar to that for ligamentous repair or prosthetic ligament replacement used in conjunction with temporary immobilisation (Diamond et al., 1999; Beever et al., 2016).

Severe shearing injuries with extensive tissue loss have traditionally been treated with open wound management and temporary stabilisation with a transarticular ESF for the first 6 weeks. This allows for formation of extensive periarticular fibrous tissue and provision of long-term joint stability. However, in some instances, instability may reoccur after the removal of the ESF and require further treatment. The transarticular ESF is usually placed after 3–5 days of open wound management, which allows time to fully assess the extent and severity of the injuries, and to explore available treatment options. Alternatively, it can be placed at the time of initial wound exploration.

Pantarsal arthrodesis is considered in severe cases where the extent of bone loss precludes restoration of joint function, and as a limb salvage procedure when other treatment options have failed. Although plate arthrodesis is usually preferred, the degree of soft tissue injury may require the use of a temporary transarticular ESF (i.e. for 12 weeks).

A reasonable outcome following management of shearing injuries should be expected. However, these are severe injuries and their management is often protracted – mean healing time of 12 weeks (Diamond et al., 1999) –, expensive, and associated with multiple complications. Most complications are related to the method of joint immobilisation (i.e. associated with the use of a bandage or a transarticular ESF) but can be treated successfully. Although some degree of long-term lameness is expected in most patients, owner satisfaction has been reported as good or excellent in several reviews of management of shearing injuries (Beardsley and Schrader, 1995; Diamond et al., 1999; Beever et al., 2016). Management of shearing injuries in cats is similar to that in dogs and the same principles apply (Corr, 2009), although less data is available for comparison.

Box 1. Management and soft tissue–healing progression of a severe shearing tarsal injury in a 6-year-old domestic shorthair cat following a road traffic accident.

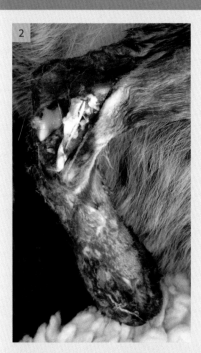

Figure 2. Lateral aspect of the distal right hindlimb showing severe trauma to the supporting structures of the tarsal joint, including lateral collateral ligament, joint capsule, lateral malleolus and lateral talar trochlear ridge. There is also a deep lateral shearing injury at the distal metatarsal and proximal phalangeal level. Note the degree of wound contamination of both wounds and the difficulty in discerning tissue viability at this stage.

Figure 3. Lateral (a) and medial (b) views of the same limb following 2 days of open wound management that included daily wound lavage and conservative tissue debridement. A large skin deficit is also present on the medial aspect of the distal tibia and tarsus. Note how debris and necrotic tissue have been removed but some areas of questionable tissue viability still remain.

Figure 4. Lateral aspect of the same limb following 6 days of open wound management. Note the presence of healthy granulation tissue covering the tarsal wound and developing on the distal one.

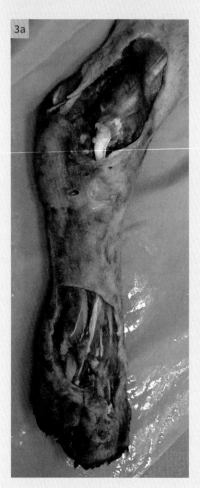

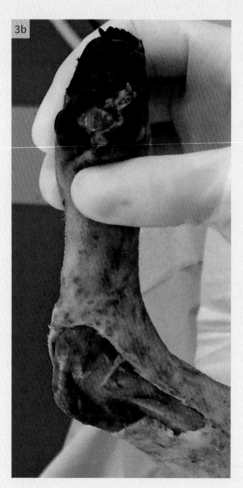

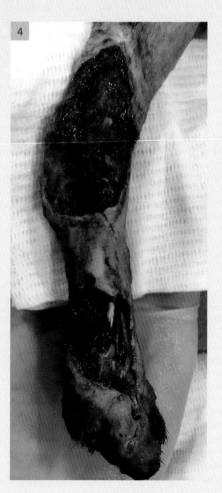

Figure 5. Lateral (a) and medial (b) views of the same limb 13 days after the initial trauma and immediately after removal of a negative pressure wound therapy (NPWT) device. Pantarsal arthrodesis with dorsal plating and simultaneous placement of a mesh skin graft around 80 % of the circumference of the hock was carried out 4 days earlier. The only viable skin around the tarsal joint at the time of arthrodesis was on the dorsal aspect, and this was used to cover the plate. Immediately after surgery a NPWT was placed for 4 days to maximise graft take and tissue viability. Graft survival was 100 %. At the time of surgery, the wound on the metatarsal/phalangeal area was not deemed suitable for grafting and, although later mesh or punch grafting was planned, the wound eventually healed by second intention.

Figure 6. Appearance of the distal wound 7 weeks after initial trauma. Epithelisation is complete, although remodelling is still ongoing on the distal wound.

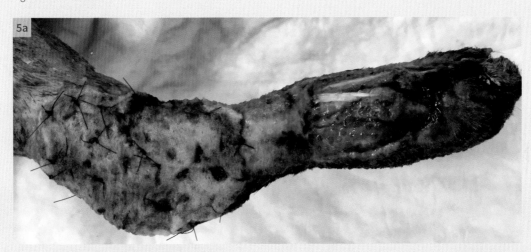

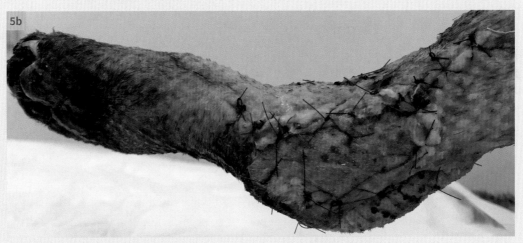

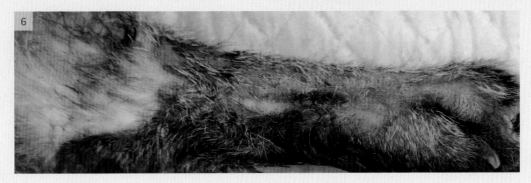

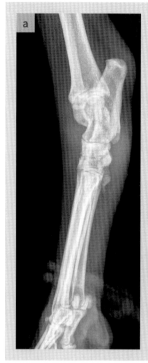
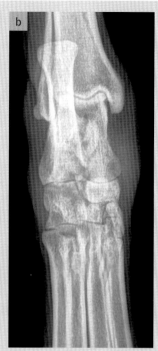
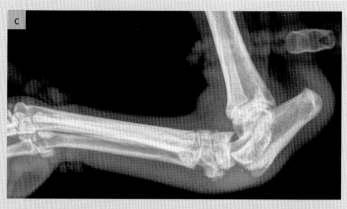

Figure 7. Preoperative mediolateral (a), dorsoplantar (b) and stressed mediolateral radiographs (c) of the right tarsal joint of a 10-year-old Shetland Sheepdog affected by severe intertarsal plantar instability. Severe soft tissue swelling can be seen associated with the unstable joint. Note the degree of joint luxation when the joint is placed under stress.

INTERTARSAL SUBLUXATION AND LUXATION

Subluxation of the calcaneoquartal and talocalcaneocentral joints is usually secondary to disruption of the plantar ligaments and is most common in Shetland Sheepdogs and other Collie-type dogs (Fig. 7). The cause is unknown. It causes progressive plantigrade stance, which is usually bilateral. This is a surgical condition and the preferred treatment is partial tarsal arthrodesis of the intertarsal and tarsometatarsal joints with a lateral plate. Previously popular alternative arthrodesis methods, such as the use of a transfixation pin or a lag screw combined with a tension-band, are significantly associated with a higher rate of major complications and clinical failure (Barnes et al., 2013).

Dorsal intertarsal instability is uncommon and is usually caused by traumatic disruption of the weak dorsal short ligaments. Conservative management with external coaptation for 6 weeks is advised; if this fails to stabilise the joint, partial tarsal arthrodesis is advised (Allan, 2014).

TARSOMETATARSAL SUBLUXATION AND LUXATION

Tarsometatarsal joint instability (Fig. 8) is uncommon and is usually caused by traumatic disruption of the dorsal or plantar ligaments. Concurrent tarsal fractures and metatarsal ligamentous avulsion fractures are common due to the inherent stability of this joint and the considerable force required to disrupt it.

Standard treatment of this condition is by partial tarsal arthrodesis of the intertarsal and tarsometatarsal joints via lateral plating. Alternative arthrodesis options include the use of a transarticular ESF, transfixation pins, intramedullary pinning or medial plating. Use of a transarticular ESF may be preferred for open wounds and medial plating for injuries with loss of bone integrity that require buttress support to the medial aspect of the joint.

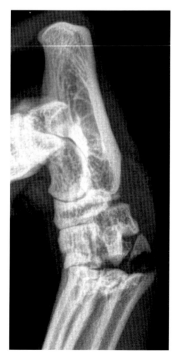

Figure 8. Stressed mediolateral radiograph of the right tarsus of a 4-year-old British Shorthair with traumatic plantar tarsometatarsal instability. Concurrent metatarsal ligamentous avulsion fractures are common, as shown in this case.

SURGICAL MANAGEMENT

MALLEOLAR FRACTURE REPAIR

Introduction

Malleolar fractures are articular fractures that require early internal rigid fixation. Treatment options include the use of one or two small parallel pins with a figure-of-eight tension-band wire, two diverging Kirschner wires or a lag screw. The choice of implant depends primarily on the size of the patient (i.e. screws for large patients). Fixation of lateral malleolar fractures is usually indirect, since the malleolar fragment is fixed to the tibia rather than the fibula.

Surgical planning

Preoperative orthogonal radiographs of the affected joint should be taken.

Surgical technique

The affected limb is clipped and aseptically prepared to include the paw and the patient is placed on the operating table in lateral recumbency with a hanging limb technique, with the affected limb uppermost if the joint is affected laterally, and lowermost if the joint is affected medially. If the injury is bilateral, the patient is positioned in dorsal recumbency.

A standard approach to the lateral or medial malleolus (Fig. 9) and talocrural joint is performed (Johnson, 2013).

A curved skin incision is made from the distal fourth of the tibia to the proximal metatarsal area, centred on the affected malleolus. The subcutis and deep crural fascia are dissected and retracted to allow for complete examination of the malleolus and collateral ligament. For lateral malleolar fractures, the saphenous vein is identified before incising the skin distally. Following dissection of the superficial and deep fascia, the extensor retinaculum is identified and transected in a line parallel to the cranial edge of the peroneus longus tendon. This allows caudal retraction of the tendon that overlies the lateral malleolus. For both medial and lateral malleolar fractures a periosteal elevator can be used to identify and dissect around the fracture line. The fragments are then reduced and the fracture repaired using a standard internal repair technique. Small point-to-point bone-holding forceps can be used to position the fragment. Due to the small size and distal location of the malleolar fragment (it can reach 1–2 cm distal to the talocrural joint), it is important to ensure that small enough Kirschner wires are used to prevent further malleolar fracture and that they are angled proximally to

avoid joint penetration. In very small patients, placement of a single pin may be the only option (Figs. 10 and 11). Recommended pin sizes include 0.9–1.1 mm for cats and small dogs and 1.6–1.9 mm for larger patients. Recommended tension-band wire sizes include 0.56–0.8 mm for cats and small dogs and 1–1.25 mm for larger patients (Bojrab et al., 2014). Following malleolar stabilisation, the wound is lavaged and closed in a routine fashion.

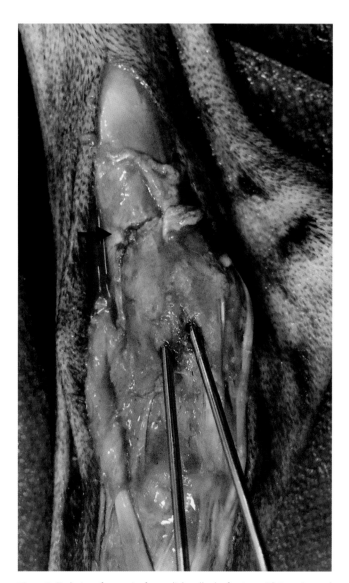

Figure 9. Technique for repair of a medial malleolar fracture with two pins and orthopaedic wire in a figure-of-eight configuration in a medium-size crossbreed dog. Following standard approach to the area, the margins of the malleolus and fracture line (arrow) are defined. This can be aided by the use of a periosteal elevator. It must be ensured that the joint is not penetrated at the time of placement of the Kirschner wires.

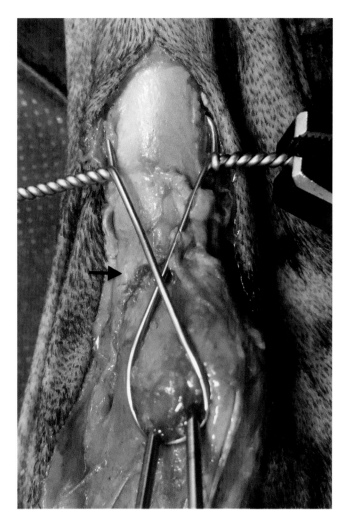 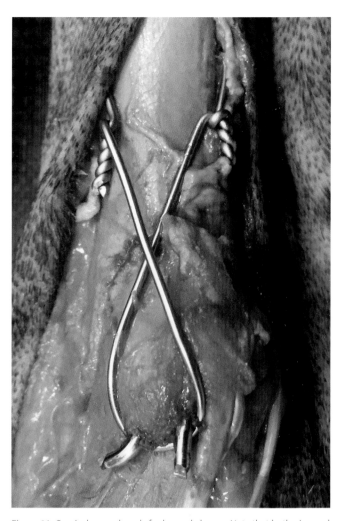

Figure 10. The transverse tibial tunnel for placement of the orthopaedic wire is roughly at the same distance from the fracture line as the entry point of the pins to the malleolus. Both ends of the orthopaedic wire are tightened simultaneously and with mild traction to ensure even tension along the tension-band.

Figure 11. Surgical wound ready for layered closure. Note that both pins and orhopaedic wire have been cut short and bent flat to prevent excessive soft tissue irritation.

Postoperative management

Malleolar repairs are protected postoperatively for 2–4 weeks. The decision between use of an orthotic device, splint, cast or transarticular ESF will depend on the strength of the repair and the presence of concurrent injuries (i.e. shearing injuries). Although the types of complications associated with each stabilisation system are different, the long-term outcomes are similar (Beever et al., 2016).

Surgical wounds are cold packed for the first 3 days and NSAIDs prescribed for 2 weeks. Radiographs are taken immediately postoperatively (Fig. 12) and 6 weeks later. The exercise is limited to lead walks for the first 8 weeks or until there is radiographic evidence of bone healing.

Outcome

The prognosis for normal function following timely repair of closed malleolar fractures (within 5–7 days of injury) is good. Degenerative joint disease may, however, still develop (Tobias and Johnston, 2013). In feline patients, poor results have been reported when bilateral instability is present in the same joint. Osteoarthritis is a common sequel of severe tarsal instability or post-traumatic joint incongruity (Schmökel et al., 1994).

Complications

Common intraoperative complications include fragmentation of the malleolus secondary to use of an oversized implant (i.e. pin or screw) and penetration of the joint space due to incorrect angulation of the implant. Postoperative complications are usually related to infection or failure of the repair.

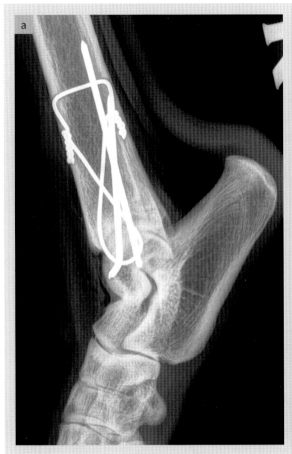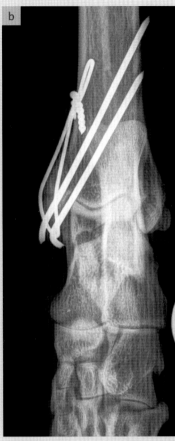

Figure 12. Postoperative mediolateral (a) and dorsoplantar (b) radiographs following repair of a medial malleolar fracture with two pins and tension-band technique. Same patient as in Figures 9–11. In this case the presence of a large malleolar fragment allowed the repair with relatively large Kirschner wires. With smaller malleolar fragments, use of smaller pins may be required. Note that the cranial pin enters the proximal fragment slightly too distal, violating the tibiotarsal joint space. In this case interference with joint function was not noted and replacement of the pin was not required. The cranial pin should also have been aimed in a more cranial direction to ensure both pins are running parallel to each other.

Temporary joint stabilisation following repair often also leads to complications, although the majority of these can be managed successfully.

TRANSARTICULAR EXTERNAL SKELETAL FIXATION IN THE TARSAL JOINT

Introduction
Standard principles of external skeletal fixation should be adhered to when this technique is applied to the tarsal joint.

Indications
Tarsal transarticular ESFs are most commonly used to provide temporary tarsal joint support during the healing process of injuries of the common calcaneal tendon and collateral ligaments, and for joint arthrodesis following severe shearing injuries.

The transarticular ESF is left in place for 3–4 weeks when used for temporary joint stabilisation following common calcaneal tendon or collateral ligament repair. Following ESF removal a splint or orthosis can be used. Hinged transarticular ESFs can be unlocked after the initial 4 weeks when used for collateral ligament repair. Transarticular ESFs used for management of severe shearing injuries are usually left for 6 weeks, to allow for periarticular fibrosis to form. When used to promote arthrodesis, the transarticular ESF is usually left in place for 12 weeks.

Surgical planning
Preoperative radiographs that include the tibia, tarsus and metatarsal bones are required for preoperative planning.

A variety of ESF configurations can be used depending on the type of patient (i.e. size and ability to rest postoperatively), intended use and expected healing time. Reported types of linear configurations used in the tarsal joint (with incremental levels of stiffness provided) include type I, type II and type IIb. Variations include the use of extra connecting bars, acrylic bars, hinged ESFs and circular ESFs. Unfortunately, the absence of mechanical studies on transarticular ESFs does not allow for evidence-based guidelines on which type of configuration is best suited for each type of indication or patient.

Surgical technique

General recommendations for the use of ESFs in the tarsal joint apply. They include the following:

■ The strength of the construct must be matched with the patient weight and temperament, time to frame removal and indication (i.e. use of a transarticular ESF for joint arthrodesis requires absolute stability for a prolonged period of time, and therefore increased ESF strength and stiffness).

■ Increased strength of the construct can be achieved by increasing pin size and number, use of full pins and use of extra connecting bars.

■ Pin size should not exceed 30 % of the bone diameter and a minimum of three pins should be used above and below the tibiotarsal joint to minimise the risk of complications, even in feline patients (Kulendra et al., 2011).

■ Positive profile pins are predrilled with a drill bit 10 % smaller than the pin and are angled perpendicular to the bone axis. Smooth pins are placed at 70 degrees to the bone.

■ Pins should be placed through "safe" soft tissue corridors and risk of thermal bone injury should be considered and avoided. Pins should not be placed closer than three times their diameter to a joint surface.

■ Hinged type I transarticular ESFs used for management of tarsocrural joint instabilities should be initially locked and can be loosened after 4 weeks to allow for controlled movement in the plane of motion of the joint while ensuring the joint remains protected from mediolateral instability (Jaeger et al., 2005).

Recommendations for feline patients are as follows:

■ Type I configurations with a minimum of three pins above and below the tibiotarsal joint are used routinely. The pins can be placed contralateral to the side of the lesion to penetrate healthy skin if required. Stiffness of the construct can easily be increased by adding an extra connecting bar in a triangular configuration. A steel connecting bar contoured to about 120 degrees can be used to connect all the pins (Fig. 13) or, alternatively, separate connecting bars are used.

■ Type II/IIb frames may be used when increased or prolonged stability is required.

■ Pin size: 1.6 mm pins are generally used in the tibia and 1.2–1.6 mm pins in the tarsal and metatarsal bones.

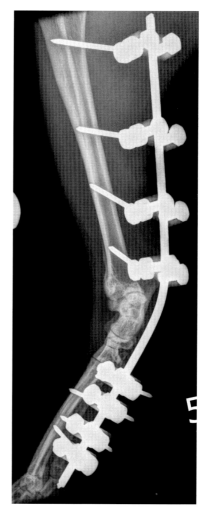

Figure 13. Immediate postoperative mediolateral radiograph of a type I transarticular external skeletal fixator (ESF) placed in a 6-year-old domestic shorthair cat for management of a shearing injury that was causing instability of the tibiotarsal joint. In this case four pins were placed both in the tibia and the metatarsal bones.

Recommendations for canine patients are as follows:

■ Type I frames with or without an extra triangulation bar can often be used to manage simpler injuries (i.e. tarsal instability).

■ Type II/IIb frames (Figs. 14 and 15) are often used in heavier patients, for injuries causing more severe joint instability and when longer healing time is expected.

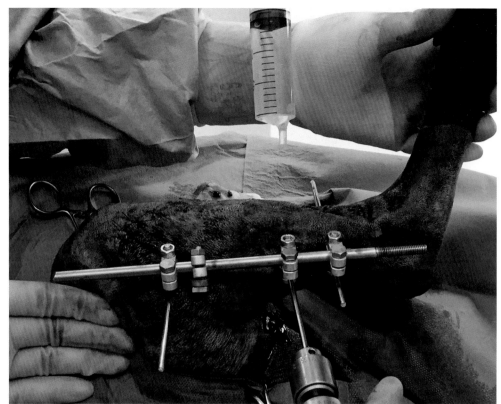

Figure 14. Placement of a hinged type IIb transarticular external skeletal fixator (ESF) for management of traumatic lateral tibiotarsal instability in a 10-year-old boxer. Placement of the tibial component of the ESF. The most distal and proximal pins and the connecting bar are already in place. Additional positive profile pins are being placed through the clamps perpendicular to the axis of the bone. Predrilling of pinholes with an appropriately sized drill bit and use of saline to prevent thermal osteonecrosis are shown.

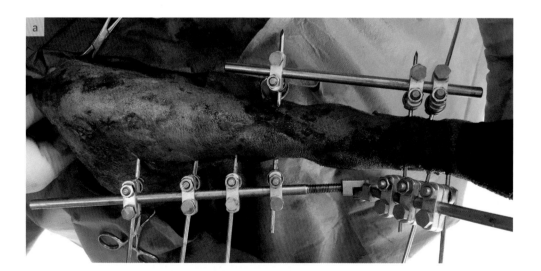

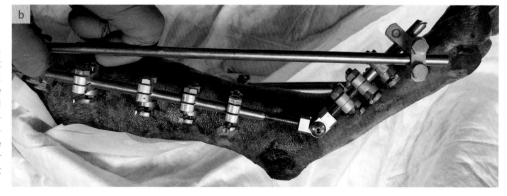

Figure 15. Cranial (a) and lateral (b) views of the limb following placement of the transarticular external skeletal fixator. A hinge has been placed on the lateral aspect of the limb and a third connecting bar is being placed in a triangular configuration following postoperative radiographs. If the hinge is to be used, the triangular configuration bar can be removed and the full pins cut short on the medial side.

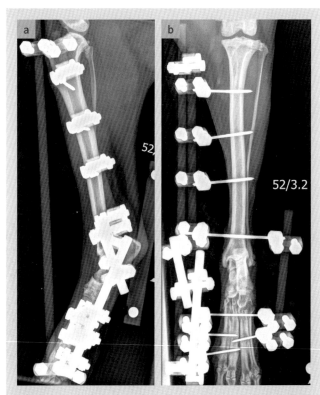

Figure 16. Follow-up mediolateral (a) and dorsoplantar (b) radiographs 4 weeks after placement of a type IIb transarticular external skeletal fixator (ESF) for management of a chronic common calcaneal tendon mechanism injury in a 9-year-old Labrador Retriever. The ESF frame placed in this case is similar to that in Figures 14 and 15. However, the tibial and metatarsal connecting bars are placed on the medial aspect and linked by a third connecting bar and double clamps, as well as by a fourth connecting bar to create the triangular configuration. Note the radiolucency and periosteal reaction associated to the most distal metatarsal pin, which was causing discomfort and discharge. The ESF was removed, and a splinted bandage was placed for another 3 weeks.

Postoperative management

Radiographs are taken immediately after surgery and at appropriate time intervals (i.e. at 6 weeks postoperatively and every 4–6 weeks thereafter). Following ESF placement, open wounds are covered with a sterile nonadherent dressing, and sterile swabs or sponges are placed around the pins and under the connecting bars. A modified Robert Jones bandage can be applied covering the entire frame and foot, and is maintained for 2–4 days to prevent excessive postoperative swelling of the distal limb. In the presence of shearing injuries, the bandage may need to be changed daily. After 2–4 days the frame should be protected with both gauze and elastic bandage. Postoperative analgesics and NSAIDs are prescribed as required. Exercise restriction, including cage/room rest and short lead walks, as well as enrolment in a physical rehabilitation programme are advised.

Routine advice applies for postoperative monitoring and cleaning of the skin–pin interface of the ESF, care of the ESF protective bandage, open wound management and follow-up examinations. Standard follow-up examinations are carried out at 10–14 days and 6 weeks postoperatively, and every 4 weeks thereafter until the frame is removed. It is important that the owner inspects the frame and skin–pin interfaces daily for evidence of increased inflammation or discharge and that any ESF-associated complications are identified and addressed promptly. A progressive increase in controlled mobilisation may be required following transarticular ESF removal and will depend on the nature of the original injury.

Outcome

Reported functional outcomes following the use of a transarticular ESF for tendon and ligament injuries, shearing wounds, fractures, luxations and arthrodeses vary from fair to excellent (Tobias and Johnston, 2013). The outcome depends predominantly on the underlying pathology.

In a retrospective study that evaluated outcome following the use of a transarticular ESF for treatment of tarsocrural instability in 32 cats, owner satisfaction was excellent in most cases. However, over half of the patients did exhibit some degree of lameness (Kulendra et al., 2011).

Complications

Complications will almost invariably occur with prolonged use of a transarticular ESF. However, by adhering to the basic principles of frame application and with the right choice of implant for each individual case, complications can be minimised.

Complications associated with the use of an ESF can be grouped in three categories (Kraus et al., 2008):
- Soft tissue impalement: muscles, nerves, tendons and vessels.
- Failure to maintain stability: catastrophic frame failure, pin breakage, pin pull-out, premature pin loosening and bone fracture.
- Infection: osteomyelitis, sequestration, major pin tract infection and minor pin tract infection.

Loosening, bending and breakage of multiple pins is suggestive of a poor technique (i.e. thermal bone necrosis) or underestimation of the strength of the frame required for the patient.

PARTIAL AND PANTARSAL ARTHRODESIS

Introduction

Pantarsal arthrodesis (PTA) is the fusion of the tarsocrural, intertarsal and tarsometatarsal joints at a functional angle. Pantarsal arthrodesis by application of a bone plate is the favoured technique when fusion of the tarsocrural joint is required, although use of a transarticular ESF may be favoured in the presence of large or infected open wounds (i.e. with shearing injuries).

Dorsal, medial, lateral and plantar techniques have been described for plate application for pantarsal arthrodesis, although medial plating is most commonly performed in dogs and dorsal plating in cats. Dorsal plating is not bio-mechanically sound and the use of dorsal plates has traditionally been reserved for smaller patients. New dorsal hybrid dynamic compression plates (HDCP) with improved design features may be a suitable alternative for larger patients, although there is no literature to support their use to date. Lateral plating may be considered in cases where the use of medial plating is precluded (i.e. medial shearing injuries); this requires distal fibular resection or displacement. Caudal plate application, although biomechanically sound, requires extensive soft tissue dissection and is not favoured routinely. Augmentation of the medial or lateral plate repair with a calcaneotibial screw is recommended in dogs. Alternative methods for augmentation of arthrodesis repair include placement of a second plate or use of intramedullary pins, a transarticular ESF or transarticular screws.

Partial tarsal arthrodesis (PaTA) is the fusion of the intertarsal and/or tarsometatarsal joints, and lateral plating is usually favoured. A medial plate can be used when the use of a lateral plate is precluded; however, it has been associated with plantar necrosis, a severe complication. Dorsal and plantar plating for PaTA have also been reported but are not routinely used.

> Central to any kind of arthrodesis is meticulous articular cartilage debridement, use of bone graft and rigid fixation.

Indications

Pantarsal arthrodesis is a salvage procedure that is indicated when other methods to preserve joint function have failed. Indications include:

- Traumatic joint injuries that are beyond repair. This includes severe shearing injuries and comminuted tarsal fractures.
- Unstable joints where alternative methods of repair have failed or are not favoured.
- Failure beyond repair of the common calcaneal tendon mechanism.
- Intractable tarsal pain, including medically nonresponsive osteoarthritis and some osteochondrosis lesions.

Partial tarsal arthrodesis is primarily indicated for the management of plantar instability of the intertarsal and tarso-metatarsal joints, and dorsal intertarsal instability not responsive to conservative management.

Surgical planning

For arthrodesis of the tarsocrural joint, achieving a functional angle is critical. This angle is usually between 135 and 145 degrees in dogs and between 115 and 125 degrees in cats. The current range of commercial pre-bent plates can be used in most patients; these include canine PTA plates with a 135- and 140-degree flexion angle, and feline plates with a 120-degree flexion angle. Alternatively, the standing angle of flexion of the affected limb can be derived from the contralateral limb and a custom-made plate can be ordered.

Multiple types of plates can be used for tarsal joint arthrodesis, although hybrid dynamic compression plates (HDCP) are usually preferred for both PTA and PaTA. Preoperative orthogonal radiographs that include the distal tibia, tarsal joint and metatarsal bones are required. Some important aspects to be considered for accurate preoperative planning include the following:

- The screw diameter should not exceed 40 % of the diameter of any bone (Johnson et al., 2005).
- Arthrodesis plates should span over 50 % of the length of the metatarsal bone.
- For PTA, a minimum of three screws must be placed in both the tibial and metatarsal bones. For dorsal PTA, a minimum of two screws should engage both the talus and the calcaneus (Johnson et al., 2005).
- For PaTA with laterally placed plates, three or more screws are placed in the calcaneus and in the metatarsal bones (two in cats), and one or two screws are placed in the

fourth tarsal bone. The distal calcaneal screw should also engage the talus (Johnson et al., 2005; Montavon et al., 2009). For PaTA with medially placed plates, one or two screws are placed in the talus, one screw engages both the central and the fourth tarsal bone and a minimum of three screws engage metatarsals II and III (Montavon et al., 2009; Swaim et al., 2015).

- Screw placement within joint spaces is avoided by appropriate plate positioning and angulation of the screws. This must be considered at the time of templating and again at the time of surgery.
- The need for augmentation of the repair at the time of arthrodesis, or following it (i.e. placement of a calcaneotibial screw, splinted bandage, or cast) must be anticipated.

Surgical technique

Common elements to pantarsal and partial tarsal arthrodesis techniques

For all PTA and PaTA procedures the entire affected limb is clipped and aseptically prepared, including the paw and digits. The patient is placed on the operating table in lateral or dorsal recumbency, depending on the surgical approach (appropriate table positioning is discussed for each of the procedures) with a hanging limb technique. Standard placement of quarter drapes and overdrape follows. The paw is covered with a sterile waterproof foot drape. If use of autologous cancellous bone graft is planned, it must be taken into consideration at the time of clipping, positioning on the operating table and draping.

Key points to a successful arthrodesis include:
- Systematic and thorough articular cartilage debridement
- Use of bone graft to promote bone fusion
- Joint compression, rigid fixation and correct limb alignment
- Preservation of blood supply and tension-free wound closure

Meticulous joint debridement (Fig. 17) is required to allow joint fusion to occur for long-term success. This is best performed with a pneumatic high-speed burr. Deep joint debridement is facilitated by manipulation of the joint (i.e. varus deviation for lateral PaTA) and use of a Freer periosteal elevator or small Hohmann retractor as a fulcrum to distract the joint. The articular cartilage is debrided down

to the subchondral bone. Excessive subchondral bone is not removed as this can delay arthrodesis. The sclerotic subchondral bone can have holes drilled through it to create vascular access channels to the medullary canal. The joint is irrigated during debridement to cool down the burr tip and prevent thermal bone necrosis.

Autogenous bone graft is most commonly harvested from the proximal metaphyseal region of the humerus (Fig. 18). Alternative donor sites include the iliac crest and the proximal tibial metaphysis. The greater tubercle of the humerus can be easily palpated on the craniolateral aspect of the proximal humerus, and mild internal rotation and stabilisation of the elbow in that position facilitates the collection of bone graft from this area. A 2–3 cm long skin incision directly over the tubercle is followed by sharp transection of the subcutis

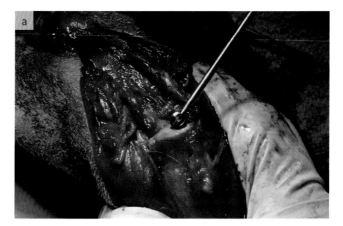

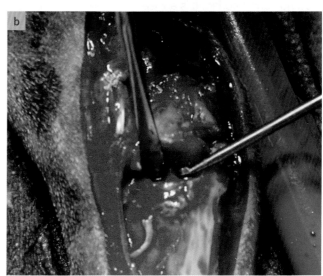

Figure 17. Technique for joint debridement prior to arthrodesis. A large burr head is used for large joints and in areas of easy access (a). A Hohmann retractor or a Freer periosteal elevator can be used to facilitate joint distraction in smaller joints and deeper areas (b). A smaller burr head is used in these areas. Joint irrigation should be used liberally during joint debridement.

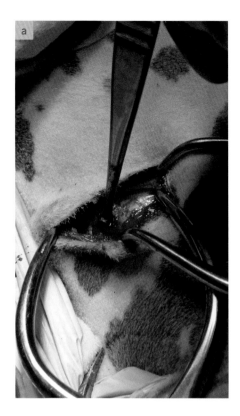
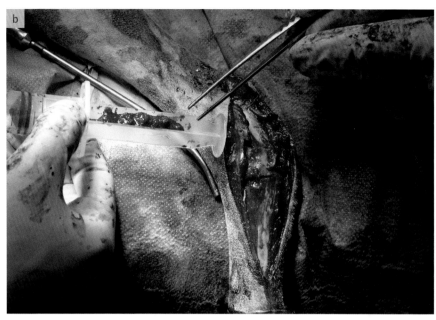

Figure 18. Process of harvesting of cancellous bone graft from the proximal humerus and application into the debrided joint to arthrodese. After gaining access into the proximal humeral metaphyseal area a small curette is being used to harvest the cancellous bone graft (a). Note how blood clots and the cancellous graft material have been collected and placed in the plunger of a syringe for immediate use (b). Immediately following collection, the graft material is packed in all joint spaces to be arthrodesed.

and deep fascia down to the level of the bone. Gelpi retractors can be placed to keep the fascia retracted. If encountered, the deltoid muscle is retracted caudally. A large cortical bone window can be opened with a burr, large drill bit or Steinmann pin. The trabecular bone is harvested with a curette and is kept in a blood-soaked swab or in the barrel of a syringe until needed. It is advised to avoid breaking down or crushing the harvested cancellous bone, to keep any collected blood clots and to use the graft material immediately after collection. The graft material should be gently and evenly packed into the debrided (and lavaged) recipient joint space/s. Any excess bone graft can be gently compressed into the joint or later packed around the plate, but crushing or excessive compaction of graft material should be avoided.

The use of cancellous bone graft is the gold standard for promotion of bone healing because it uses all the strategies of bone regeneration. However, harvesting of graft material causes morbidity, and it must be used immediately after collection as cell viability decreases very rapidly. Alternatively, the use of powdered demineralised bone matrix combined with cancellous bone (commercially available), particularly when a source of progenitor cells is added (i.e. whole blood or bone marrow), can be equally effective in promoting bone healing (Hoffer et al., 2008).

Advice for plating includes the following:

- For lateral and medial arthrodesis, plate contouring is facilitated by performing it before joint debridement (i.e. on the stable joint) and after gentle burring of any bony prominences of the surface to be plated (i.e. protuberances at the base of metatarsal V, the calcaneus and the fourth tarsal bone for lateral PaTA).
- The plate must be contoured in the same position as planned preoperatively (i.e. so that plate holes do not overlie joints) and very slightly over-contoured at the level of the arthrodesis to prevent postoperative valgus or varus deviation for lateral and medial arthrodesis respectively.
- At the time of plating it is critical to ensure appropriate limb alignment and that all screw holes are centred in their respective bones, particularly along the smaller metatarsal bones, to prevent bone fractures.
- Correct positioning of the crucial first screw can be facilitated by marking the correct location through the plate with electrocautery, removing the plate and focusing on placing the drill in the centre of the bone and with the appropriate angulation.
- The use of hypodermic needles or small Kirschner wires facilitates the location of joints and cortical boundaries of metatarsal and tibial bones to ensure that screw holes are centred in their respective bones.

- Placement of screws between joints must be avoided (i.e. calcaneoquartal joint), although intertarsal joint impingement is not associated with lameness. Screws should be angled away from joints as necessary.
- Screws in the metatarsal bones for lateral and medial arthrodesis should engage fewer metatarsal bones as they become more distal. The most proximal screw should engage four metatarsal bones, the following screw three, the next one two and the most distal screw only one metatarsal bone. There is more movement between metatarsal bones as they become more distal and it is very common for distal metatarsal screws to become loose or for metatarsal bones to fracture if a distal screw engages three or four metatarsal bones.
- Use of loaded screws allows for compression of the joint space to facilitate arthrodesis, although only one compression screw per joint level is advised to prevent any joint deviation (i.e. valgus deviation for PaTA with lateral plating; Johnson et al., 2005).
- Soft tissues should be handled gently, blood supply preserved and wound closure tension-free; tension-free closure may require a combination of undermining, tension-relieving sutures and relaxing incisions.

Partial tarsal arthrodesis, lateral approach

The patient is positioned for surgery in lateral recumbency with the affected limb uppermost. A standard lateral approach to the tarsal joint is performed, extending from the proximal calcaneus to the mid-metatarsal area (Fig. 19) (Johnson, 2013). The skin incision is followed by a combination of blunt and sharp dissection of the subcutaneous and deep fascia along the same line of incision. The sharp incision to the deep fascia is made dorsal to the metatarsal vessels to allow for their plantar retraction. Contouring of the plate is facilitated by the sharp excision of the lateral collateral ligament and joint capsule, and by burring of any bony prominences. Once the plate is contoured the articular cartilage is debrided at the level of the calcaneoquartal and fifth, fourth and third tarsometatarsal joints. The joints are thoroughly lavaged and the bone graft is packed into them.

Plating is started by placement of a distal metatarsal screw and followed by placement of a proximal calcaneal and fourth tarsal bone screws. The most distal calcaneal screw should engage the talus and the screw in the fourth tarsal bone should span the entire tarsus below the proximal intertarsal joint (Fig. 20). Closure of the wound is performed in a routine fashion.

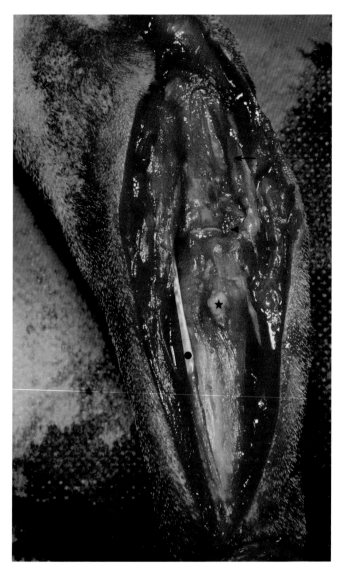

Figure 19. Lateral approach to the tarsal joint for partial tarsal arthrodesis (PaTA) with lateral plating in a 10-year-old Shetland Sheepdog. Preoperative radiographs of this case can be seen in Figure 7. Following skin incision and dissection of the subcutaneous and deep fascia, the following anatomical landmarks can be identified (plantar is to the right): tendon of the peroneus longus (circle), insertion of the long part of the lateral collateral ligament, excised (star), tarsometatarsal joint (arrowhead) and level of calcaneoquartal joint (arrow). Following burring of any bony prominences, templating of the bone can be carried out in preparation for plating.

Partial tarsal arthrodesis, medial approach

The patient is positioned for surgery in lateral recumbency with the affected limb lowermost. A standard medial approach to the tarsal joint is made from the proximal talus to the mid-metatarsal level (Johnson et al., 2005). The skin incision is followed by a combination of blunt and sharp dissection of the subcutaneous and deep fascia along the same line of incision. Excision of the medial collateral ligament and joint capsule and gentle burring of any bony prominences in the area facilitates the contouring of the plate, ensuring that

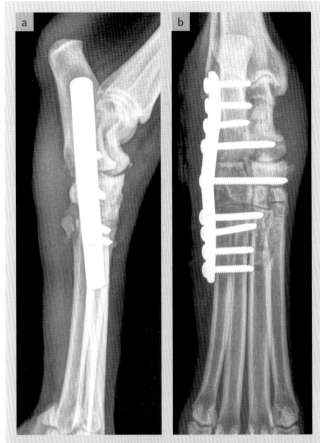

Figure 20. Postoperative mediolateral (a) and dorsoplantar (b) radiographs following partial tarsal arthrodesis with lateral plating. Same patient as in Figure 7. Note that the most distal calcaneal screw engages the talus, the next screw down engages both fourth and central tarsal bones and all metatarsal screws engage a minimum of four cortices. However, several screws could be longer to increase bone purchase.

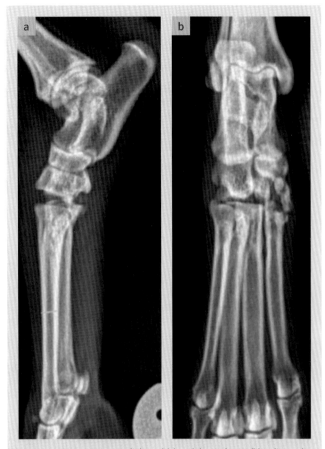

Figure 21. Preoperative mediolateral (a) and dorsoplantar (b) radiographs showing avulsion fracture of the second metatarsal bone and suspected loss of buttress support of the medial aspect of the joint in a 6-year-old Cocker Spaniel.

the plate is in the same position as planned preoperatively (Figs. 21–23). The articular cartilage is debrided at the level of the intertarsal and tarsometatarsal joints. This is followed by joint lavage and placement of the bone graft before medial plating. The first plate screw is placed through the distal metatarsals II and III, followed by the screws in the proximal talus, central and fourth tarsal bones, and finally the remaining screws (Fig. 24). Closure is routine.

Pantarsal arthrodesis, medial approach

The patient is positioned for surgery in lateral recumbency with the affected limb lowermost. A standard medial approach is made to the tarsal joint, extending from the distal third of the tibia to the middle of the second metatarsal bone; the incision is similar in length to the plate. Following skin incision, the subcutaneous and deep fasciae are transected along the same line.

The medial malleolus is burred flat and the periarticular soft tissues (joint capsule and medial collateral ligament) are excised sharply to facilitate contouring of the pre-bent plate, which is positioned as planned preoperatively (Fig. 25). Electing to drill and loosely place some screws before joint debridement may help prevent alignment or torsional deformities and can be done at this stage (Figs. 26 and 27).

The plate is then removed and the joint spaces are exposed from distal to proximal to facilitate joint debridement. The joint spaces are lavaged and the bone graft is placed. The following order of screws has been reported to secure the plate: the first screw is centred in the talus and this is followed by the central/fourth tarsal bone screw if using a plate with a T4 slot (Figs. 28 and 29). The remaining screws can be placed in the following order: proximal metatarsal, distal metatarsal, remaining metatarsal, distal tibial and remaining tibial screws (McKee et al., 2004). Joint compression can be performed as previously described (see "Advice for plating", p. 103).

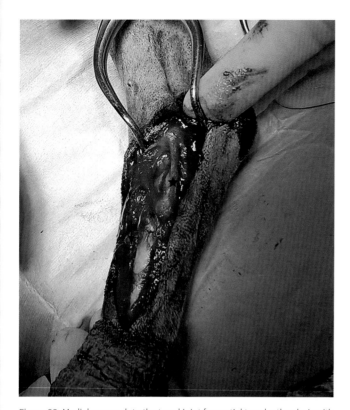

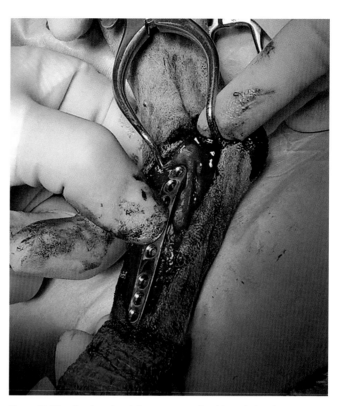

Figure 22. Medial approach to the tarsal joint for partial tarsal arthrodesis with medial plating. Following skin incision and dissection of the subcutaneous tissue along the same line, the following anatomical landmarks can be identified (plantar is to the right): long component of the medial collateral ligament (star), which inserts distally onto the central and first tarsal bones; tendon of insertion of the cranial tibial muscle (asterisk), which reaches the plantar surface of the base of metatarsal bones I and II; and metatarsal II, which can be clearly seen. The arrow follows the trajectory of the cranial tibial artery and dorsal pedal branch, which must be preserved during the soft tissue dissection.

Figure 23. The plate has already been contoured and is ready for placement.

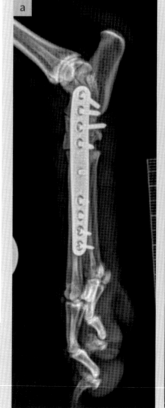
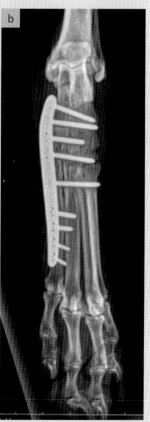

Figure 24. Postoperative mediolateral (a) and dorsoplantar (b) radiographs. The implants are correctly positioned, with two screws on the talus, one on the central tarsal bone, another on the distal row of tarsal bones and five on the metatarsal bones. A more dorsal angulation of the metatarsal screws would have allowed engaging more bone cortices per screw and therefore increased strength of the repair.

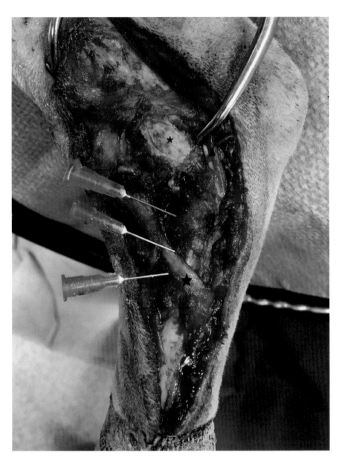

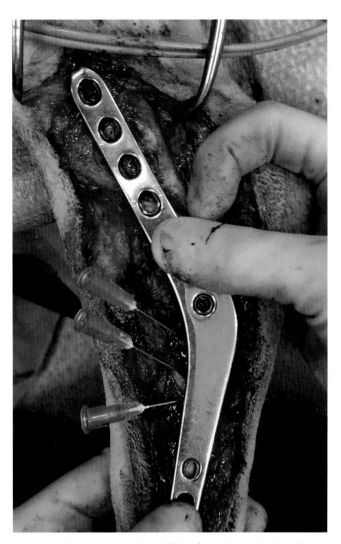

Figure 25. Medial approach to the tarsal joint of an 11-year-old German Shepherd for pantarsal arthrodesis (PTA) with medial plating. Following initial skin incision and fascial dissection, the following landmarks can be identified: medial malleolus (asterisk), that has been burred flat in preparation for plate contouring (the medial collateral ligament has been excised); the neck of the talus at the level of the proximal needle; the tendon of insertion of the cranial tibial muscle (star) between the middle and distal needles; the tarsometatarsal joint at the level of the distal needle; and the tendon of the deep digital flexor coursing distally along the plantar aspect of the joint (arrowhead).

Figure 26. Plate contouring and predrilling of several screw holes. Following initial dissection and burring of bony prominences, the plate is contoured and trialled.

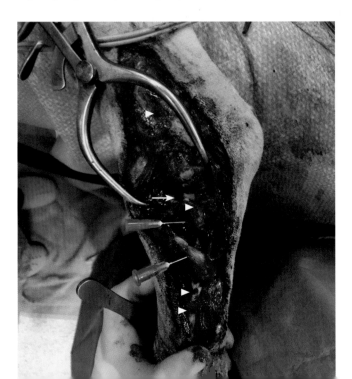

Figure 27. Several screw holes have now been drilled (arrowheads) on the distal tibia, talus and proximal metatarsal bones and the plate has once again been removed. This is now ready for joint debridement and placement of the bone graft before definitive placement of the plate. The talocrural joint and medial trochlear ridge can be seen (arrow). The needles have been replaced and are now inserted into the talocentral joint proximally and tarsometatarsal joint distally.

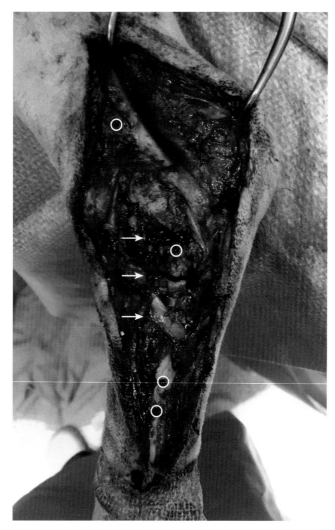

Figure 28. Grafting and plating. The talocrural and intertarsal joints have been debrided and can now be grafted. The three levels of the tarsal joint are indicated with arrows. The tarsometatarsal joint is stable and has not been disturbed. The previously drilled screw holes are also outlined (circles).

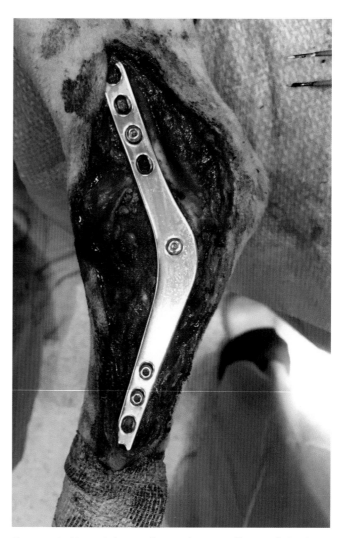

Figure 29. Grafting and plating. Following placement of bone graft, the plate is replaced, predrilled screws secured and remaining screw holes filled. This is followed by placement of a calcaneotibial screw.

Debridement of the tarsometatarsal joint can be omitted if the joint is stable preoperatively. This is because the reported incidence of postoperative plantar necrosis following medial plating when this joint is debrided is high (Roch et al., 2008). However, this surgical step is still necessary if tarsometatarsal ligamentous injury is suspected preoperatively. If debrided, ensure that the distal branches of the cranial tibial artery are preserved (see *Introduction* at the beginning of the chapter).

Partial tarsal arthrodesis with medial plating in dogs should be augmented with a calcaneotibial screw (see section *Chronic common calcaneal tendon mechanism injury*, p. 85 for a detailed description of the technique). The surgical wound is closed in a routine fashion and postoperative radiographs are taken (Fig. 30).

Pantarsal arthrodesis, dorsal approach

The patient is positioned for surgery in dorsal recumbency. A dorsomedial approach to the tarsus is made, extending from the distal fourth of the tibia to the mid-metatarsal level. Blunt dissection of the subcutis and transection of the crural extensor retinaculum allows medial retraction of the tendon of the cranial tibial muscle and cranial tibial artery and lateral retraction of the tendons of the long digital extensor muscle. It is important to preserve the dorsal pedal branch of the cranial tibial artery and its distal extension as a perforating branch between metatarsal bones II and III, particularly when debriding the tarsometatarsal joint and elevating soft tissues from metatarsal III (Figs. 31–33). Meticulous joint debridement and packing of the joint spaces with cancellous bone graft follows (Fig. 34–36).

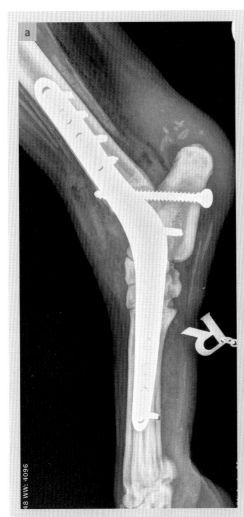

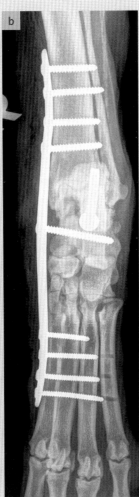

Figure 30. Postoperative mediolateral (a) and dorsoplantar (b) radiographs showing correct placement of the medial pantarsal arthrodesis plate and a calcaneotibial cortical screw and washer. Note the presence of chronic changes and soft tissue swelling associated with the common calcaneal tendon.

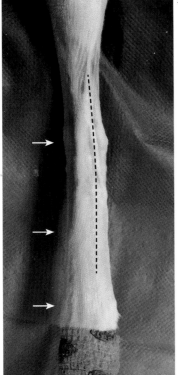

◀ Figure 31. Limb of a 5-year-old Siamese cat prepared for pantarsal arthrodesis with dorsal plating (medial is to the right) with the suggested line of skin incision. The approximate location of the tibiotarsal, tarsometatarsal and metatarsophalangeal joints is indicated (arrows).

Figure 32. Dorsal approach to the tarsal joint. Following skin incision and fascial dissection the following landmarks can be identified: tendons of the long digital extensor (star) and cranial tibial (square) muscles, crural extensor retinaculum (arrowhead), cranial tibial artery (white arrow) and its distal prolongation as dorsal pedal artery (dotted line). The dorsal pedal artery gives a distal perforating branch that disappears between metatarsals II and III (black dot). For orientation purposes the level of the talar neck has been marked with a black arrow. ▶

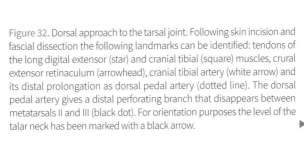

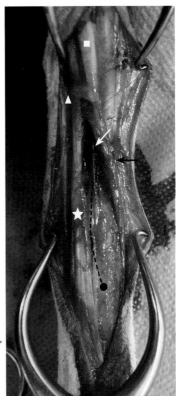

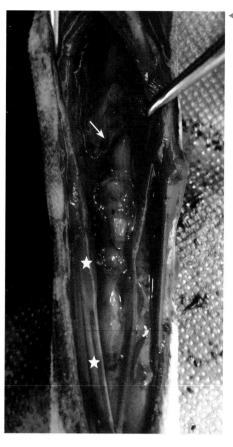

◀ Figure 33. The joint can be now identified following dissection and retraction of soft tissues. The talar ridges, and talocalcaneocentral and tarsometatarsal joints can be clearly identified (arrow and stars, respectively)

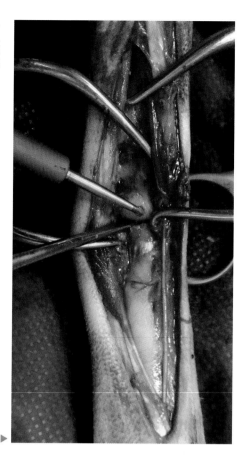

Figure 34. Joint debridement. A periosteal elevator is used to facilitate joint distraction and burring of the articular cartilage. ▶

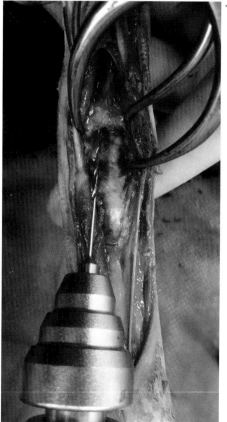

◀ Figure 35. Following standard joint debridement, osteostixis is being performed using a 1.1 mm drill bit to open vascular access channels between the distal tibial metaphysis and the talocrural joint in the presence of sclerotic subchondral bone.

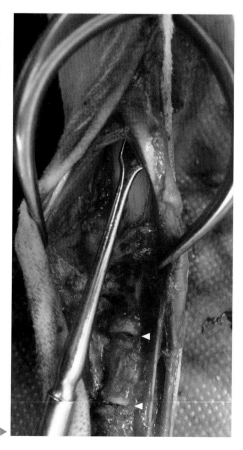

Figure 36. Creation of an epiperiosteal tunnel with a periosteal elevator to facilitate placement of the plate under the soft tissues of the distal tibia. The talocalcaneocentral and tarsometatarsal joints have now also been debrided (arrowheads) and all the joints are ready for grafting. ▶

At the time of plate placement it is important to ensure that the plate bend lies on bone at the level of the junction of the talar ridges with the talar neck. The first two screws can be placed in the third metatarsal bone and this can be followed by placement of a proximal tibial screw after correct alignment of the plate and limb are confirmed. Joints can be compressed as previously described. The two screws closest to the plate bend are angled to engage the calcaneus (Figs. 37–39). Closure of the subcutaneous tissues and skin is done in a standard fashion.

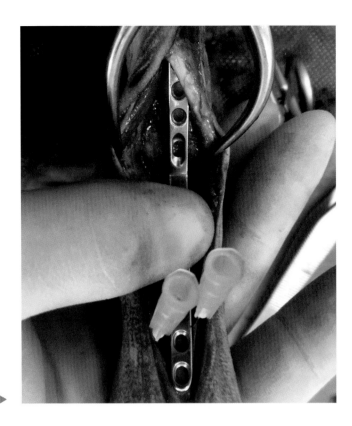

Figure 37. Plating. Correct limb alignment is being assessed in order to prevent mediolateral or torsional deformities. Hypodermic needles can be used to ensure the plate is centred within the confines of the tibial and metatarsal bones. The elbow of the plate is confirmed to sit at the appropriate level. ▶

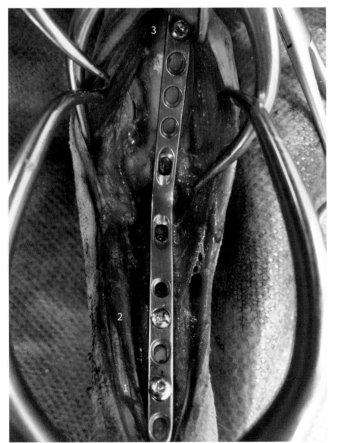

Figure 38. The order of the first three screws placed in this case is shown. Before the first tibial screw is placed bone-holding forceps can be used to temporarily secure the proximal plate to the bone and confirm once again correct limb alignment.

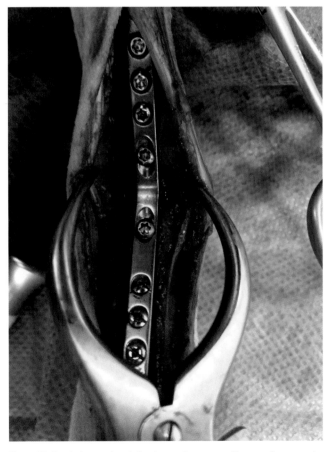

Figure 39. Surgical wound ready for closure. Any excess of bone graft can now be packed over the joint around the plate.

Postoperative management for arthrodesis procedures

Following surgery, postoperative orthogonal radiographs are obtained and a modified Robert Jones bandage is applied (Fig. 40). After 2–5 days, the soft bandage is removed and the wound is checked. Augmentation of the repair with a splinted bandage or a cast (i.e. bivalve) may be considered in some cases. However, it is currently unclear whether coaptation significantly reduces the loading on the implants and improved design may negate the need for their use. Splints and casts, if used, should be checked weekly.

Nonsteroidal anti-inflammatory drugs are prescribed for 2 weeks and owners are instructed to cage/room rest and lead exercise the patient until there is radiological evidence of fusion. Follow-up radiographs are performed every 6–8 weeks to evaluate progression of the arthrodesis, which usually takes 2–3 months. Progressive increase of exercise is usually advised for another 2-3 months. Rehabilitation therapy may be advised to overcome muscle atrophy and stiffness of the limb.

Outcome of arthrodesis

A good clinical outcome is expected in 50 to 70 % of PTA cases and in the majority of PaTA cases for as long as the principles of arthrodesis are followed and exercise restriction is ensured until radiological evidence of bone fusion.

Owners must however understand that arthrodesis is a salvage procedure with potential severe complications despite the expected good to excellent outcome in most patients. Furthermore, some degree of permanent altered gait is expected for patients undergoing pantarsal arthrodesis.

Complications of arthrodesis

Potential complications following tarsal arthrodesis with bone plates include persistent lameness, angular and rotational deformity, displacement of metatarsal bones, implant failure, bone fracture, distal limb swelling and wound-associated complications, including infection, dehiscence and plantar necrosis. Wound complications can be associated with the arthrodesis, postoperative coaptation or both.

Overall complication rates reported in multiple case series in the last 30 years range from 25 % to 80 % (Tobias and Johnston, 2013). Most procedures performed in those series were PaTA with lateral plating and PTA with medial plating. In a recent review of complications following various tarsal

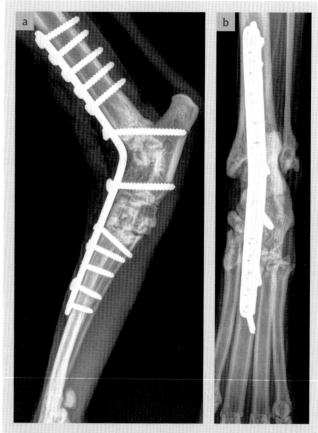

Figure 40. Postoperative mediolateral (a) and dorsoplantar (b) radiographs of the patient from Figures 31–39. Note that the screw just proximal to the plate bend engages the tibia, talus and calcaneus and the one just distal to the plate bend engages the talus and calcaneus. Also note the correct positioning of the plate and limb alignment. The most proximal metatarsal screw has been intentionally aimed distally to avoid entering the tarsometatarsal joint space.

arthrodesis procedures, intraoperative complications were recorded in 30 % of cases and postoperative complications in 75 %, with a median time of onset of 22 days. Major complications were recorded in 32 % of cases (Roch et al., 2008). The most common intraoperative complications were torsional limb deformities and metatarsal bone displacement due to failure to engage the drilled hole with the screw. Both complications can lead to long-term lameness. Pantarsal arthrodesis has a higher reported complication rate than partial arthrodesis. A major complication rate of 17 % and a 5 % clinical failure rate have been reported for PaTA with lateral plating (Barnes et al., 2013).

Morbidity associated with external coaptation following either PaTA or PTA is reported in 40 to 56 % of dogs (Roch et al., 2008; Meeson et al., 2011).

REFERENCES

CHAPTER 1

ANDERSON A, Treatment of hip dysplasia, *Journal of Small Animal Practice,* 2011, 52:182–189.

ASH K et al., Correction of craniodorsal coxofemoral luxation in cats and small breed dogs using a modified Knowles technique with the braided polyblend TightRope systems, *Veterinary and Comparative Orthopaedics and Traumatology,* 2012, 25:54–60.

BALTZER WI et al., Biomechanical analysis of suture anchors and suture materials used for toggle pin stabilization of hip joint luxation in dogs, *American Journal of Veterinary Research,* 2001, 62:721–728.

BASHER AVP, WALTER MC, NEWTON CD, Coxofemoral luxation in the dog and cat, *Veterinary Surgery,* 1986, 15:356–362.

BENNET D, DUFF SR, Transarticular pinning as a treatment for hip luxation in the dog and cat, *Journal of Small Animal Practice,* 1980, 21:373–379.

BERZON JL et al. A retrospective study of the efficacy of femoral head and neck excisions in 94 dogs and cats, 1980, *Veterinary Surgery,* 9:88–92.

BONE DL, WALKER M, CANTWELL HD, Traumatic coxofemoral luxation in dogs results of repair, *Veterinary Surgery,* 1984, 13:263–270.

CULP WT et al., Evaluation of the Norberg angle threshold: a comparison of Norberg angle and distraction index as measures of coxofemoral degenerative joint disease susceptibility in seven breeds of dogs, *Veterinary Surgery,* 2006, 35:453–459.

DECAMP CE et al., The hip joint, In: *Brinker, Piermattei and Flo's Handbook of Small Animal Orthopedics and Fracture Repair,* 5th ed., Saint Louis, Elsevier-Saunders, Saint Louis, 2016, pp. 468–517.

DEMKO JL et al., Toggle rod stabilization for treatment of hip joint luxation in dogs: 62 cases (2000–2005), *Journal of the American Veterinary Medical Association,* 2006, 229:984–989.

DOUGLAS IH, Modified De Vita pinning technique for the management of canine hip luxation: preliminary findings, *Australian Veterinary Journal,* 2000, 78:538–542.

DUFF SR, BENNETT D, Hip luxation in small animals: an evaluation of some methods of treatment, *Veterinary Record,* 1982, 111:140–143.

DUFF R, CAMPBELL JR, Long term results of excision arthroplasty of the canine hip, *The Veterinary Record,* 1977, 101:181–184.

EVERS P et al., Long-term results of treatment of traumatic coxofemoral joint dislocation in dogs: 64 cases (1973–1992), *Journal of the American Veterinary Medical Association,* 1997, 210:59–64.

FLYNN MF et al., Biomechanical evaluation of a toggle pin technique for management of coxofemoral luxation, *Veterinary Surgery,* 1994, 23:311–321.

FOX SM, Coxofemoral luxations in dogs, *Compendium of Continuing Education for the Practicing Veterinarian,* 1991, 13:381–389.

HUNT CA, HENRY WB, Transarticular pinning for repair of hip dislocation in the dog: a retrospective study of 40 cases, *Journal of the American Veterinary Medical Association,* 1985, 187:828–833.

JEFFERY ND, Femoral head and neck excision complicated by ischiatic nerve entrapment in two dogs, *Veterinary and Comparative Orthopaedics and Traumatology,* 1993, 6:215–218.

JESSEN CR, SPURRELL FA, Radiographic detection of canine hip dysplasia in known age groups, In: *Proceedings of the Canine Hip Dysplasia Symposium and Workshop,* 1972, St Louis, Mo., pp. 93–100.

JHA S, KOWALESKI MP, Mechanical analysis of twelve toggle suture constructs for stabilization of coxofemoral luxations, *Veterinary Surgery,* 2012, 41:948–953.

JOHNSON KA, *Piermattei's Atlas of Surgical Approaches to the Bones and Joints of the Dog and Cat,* 5th ed., Saint Louis, Elsevier-Saunders, 2014, pp. 322–349.

KIEVES NR et al., Hip toggle stabilization using the TightRope® system in 17 dogs: technique and long-term outcome, *Veterinary Surgery,* 2014, 43:515–522.

KNOWLES AT, KNOWLES JO, KNOWLES RP, An operation to preserve the continuity of the hip joint, *Journal of the American Veterinary Medical Association,* 1953, 123:508–515.

LEE R, FRY PD, Some observations of the occurrence of Legg-Calvé-Perthes disease (coxa plana) in the dog, and an evaluation of excision arthroplasty as a method of treatment, *Journal of Small Animal Practice,* 1969, 10:309–317.

LISKA WD et al., Total hip replacement in three cats: surgical technique, short-term outcome and comparison to femoral head ostectomy, *Veterinary and Comparative Orthopaedics and Traumatology,* 2009, 22:505–510.

MARTINI FM, SIMONAZZI B, DEL BUE M, Extra-articular absorbable suture stabilization of coxofemoral luxation in dogs *Veterinary Surgery,* 2001, 30:468–75.

McCartney W, Kiss K, McGovern F, Treatment of 70 dogs with traumatic hip luxation using a modified transarticular pinning technique, *Veterinary Record*, 2011, 168:355.

McLaughlin RM Jr, Traumatic joint luxations in small animals, *The Veterinary Clinics of North America: Small Animal Practice*, 1995, 25: 1175–1196.

Mehl NB, A new method of surgical treatment of hip dislocation in dogs and cats *Journal of Small Animal Practice*, 1988, 29:789–795.

Meij BP, Hazewinkel AW, Nap RC, Results of extra-articular stabilisation following open reduction of coxofemoral luxations in dogs and cats, *Journal of Small Animal Practice*, 1992, 33:320–326.

O'Donnell MD et al., Use of computed tomography to compare two femoral head and neck excision ostectomy techniques as performed by two novice veterinarians, *Veterinary and Comparative Orthopaedics and Traumatology*, 2015, 28:295–300.

Off W, Matis U, Resektionsarthroplastik des Hüftgelenkes bei Hunden und Katzen. Klinische, röntgenologische und ganganalytische Erhebungen an der Chirurgischen Tierklinik der Ludwig-Maximilians-Universität München, *Tierärztliche Praxis*, 1997, 25:379–387.

Ormrod AN, Treatment of hip lamenesses in the dog by excision of the femoral head, *The Veterinary Record*, 1961, 73:576–577.

Penwick RC, The variables that influence the success of femoral head and neck excision in dogs, *Veterinary Medicine*, 1992, 87:325–333.

Piek CJ et al., Long term follow-up of avascular necrosis of the femoral head in the dog, *Journal of Small Animal Practice*, 1996, 37:12–18.

Pratesi A, Grierson J, Moores AP, Toggle rod stabilisation of coxofemoral luxation in 14 cats, *Journal of Small Animal Practice*, 2012, 53:260–266.

Rawson EA, Aronsohn MG, Burk RL, Simultaneous bilateral femoral head and neck ostectomy for the treatment of canine hip dysplasia, *Journal of the American Animal Hospital Association*, 2005, 41:166–170.

Rochat M, Open reduction of coxofemoral luxations, In: *Complications in Small Animal Surgery*, Griffon D, Hamaide A, (eds.), 2016, Wiley Blackwell, Chichester, pp. 845–856.

Shani J, Johnston DE, Shahar R, Stabilization of traumatic coxofemoral luxation with an extra-capsular suture from the greater trochanter to the origin of the rectus femoris, *Veterinary and Comparative Orthopaedics and Traumatology*, 2004, 17:12–16.

Sissener TR, Whitelock RG, Langley-Hobbs SJ, Long-term results of transarticular pinning for surgical stabilisation of coxofemoral luxation in 20 cats, *Journal of Small Animal Practice*, 2009, 50:112–117.

Smith GK et al., Pathogenesis, diagnosis, and control of canine hip dysplasia, In: *Veterinary Surgery Small Animal: Volume I,* Tobias KM, Johnston SA (eds.), 2012, Elsevier-Saunders, Saint Louis, pp. 824–848.

Spreull JSA, Excision arthroplasty as a method of treatment of hip joint diseases in the dog, *The Veterinary Record*, 1961, 73:573–576.

Thacker C, Schrader SC, Caudal ventral hip luxation in the dog: a review of 14 cases, *Journal of the American Animal Hospital Association*, 1985, 21:167–172.

Towle HA, Breur GJ, Miscellaneous orthopedic conditions, In: *Veterinary Surgery Small Animal: Volume I,* Tobias KM, Johnston SA (eds.), 2012, Elsevier-Saunders, Saint Louis, pp. 1112–1126.

Wardlaw JL, McLaughlin R, Coxofemoral luxation, In: *Veterinary Surgery Small Animal: Volume I,* Tobias KM, Johnston SA (eds.), 2012, Elsevier-Saunders, Saint Louis, pp. 816–823.

Wong WT, Femoral head and neck excision, In: *Complications in Small Animal Surgery*, Griffon D, Hamaide A (eds.), 2016, Wiley Blackwell, Chichester, pp. 753–758.

Yap FW et al., Femoral head and neck excision in cats: medium- to long-term functional outcome in 18 cats, *Journal of Feline Medicine and Surgery*, 2015, 17:704–710.

CHAPTER 2

Aiken SW, Kass PH, Toombs JP, Intercondylar notch width in dogs with and without cranial cruciate ligament injuries, *Veterinary and Comparative Orthopaedics and Traumatology,* 1995, 8:128–132.

Aisa J et al., Mechanical comparison of loop and crimp configurations for extracapsular stabilization of the cranial cruciate ligament-deficient stifle, *Veterinary Surgery*, 2015, 44(1):50–58.

Apelt D et al., Effect of cranial tibial closing wedge angle on tibial subluxation: an ex vivo study, *Veterinary Surgery*, 2010, 39(4):454–459.

Aragon CL, Budsberg SC, Applications of evidence-based medicine: cranial cruciate ligament injury repair in the dog, *Veterinary Surgery*, 2005, 34(2):93–98.

ARNAULT F et al., Diagnostic value of ultrasonography to assess stifle lesions in dogs after cranial cruciate ligament rupture: 13 cases, *Veterinary and Comparative Orthopaedics and Traumatology,* 2009, 22:479–485.

ARNOCZKY SP et al., The over-the-top procedure: a technique for anterior cruciate ligament substitution in the dog, *Journal of the American Animal Hospital Association,* 1979, 15:283–290.

BARKOWSKI VJ, EMBLETON NA, Surgical technique and initial clinical experience with a novel extracapsular articulating implant for treatment of the canine cruciate ligament deficient stifle joint, *Veterinary Surgery,* 2016, 45(6):804–815.

BARRETT E et al., A retrospective study of the MRI findings in 18 dogs with stifle injuries, *Journal of Small Animal Practice,* 2009, 50:448–455.

BELL JC, NESS MG, Does use of a jig influence the precision of tibial plateau leveling osteotomy surgery? *Veterinary Surgery,* 2007 36(3):228–233.

BERGER B et al., Long-term outcome after surgical treatment of cranial cruciate ligament rupture in small breed dogs, *Tierärztliche Praxis. Ausgabe K, Kleintiere/Heimtiere,* 2015, 43:373–380.

BERGH MS, RAJALA-SCHULTZ P, JOHNSON KA, Risk factors for tibial fracture after tibial plateau leveling osteotomy in dogs, *Veterinary Surgery,* 2008, 37(4):374–382.

BERGH MS, PEIRONE B, Complications of tibial plateau levelling osteotomy in dogs, *Veterinary and Comparative Orthopaedics and Traumatology,* 2012, 25:349–358.

BLOND L et al., Diagnostic accuracy of magnetic resonance imaging for meniscal tears in dogs affected with naturally occurring cranial cruciate ligament rupture, *Veterinary Radiology and Ultrasound,* 2008, 49:425–431.

BODDEKER J et al., Computer-assisted gait analysis of the dog: comparison of two surgical techniques for the ruptured cranial cruciate ligament, *Veterinary and Comparative Orthopaedics and Traumatology,* 2012, 25:11–21.

BÖTTCHER P et al., Value of low-field magnetic resonance imaging in diagnosing meniscal tears in the canine stifle: a prospective study evaluating sensitivity and specificity in naturally occurring cranial cruciate ligament deficiency with arthroscopy as the gold standard, *Veterinary Surgery,* 2010, 39(3):296–305.

BUOTE N et al., Age, tibial plateau angle, sex and weight as risk factors for contralateral rupture of the cranial cruciate ligament in Labradors, *Veterinary Surgery,* 2009, 38(4):481–489.

BUTLER JR et al., The effects of a novel lateral extracapsular suture system on the kinematics of the cranial cruciate deficient canine stifle, *Veterinary and Comparative Orthopaedics and Traumatology,* 2013, 26:271–279.

CAMPBELL CA et al., Severity of patellar luxation and frequency of concomitant cranial cruciate ligament rupture in dogs: 162 cases (2004–2007), *Journal of the American Veterinary Medical Association,* 2010, 236:887–891.

CAREY K et al., Radiographic and clinical changes of the patellar tendon after tibial plateau leveling osteotomy 94 cases (2000–2003), *Veterinary and Comparative Orthopaedics and Traumatology,* 2005, 18:235–242.

CARPENTER DH, COOPER RC, Mini review of canine stifle joint anatomy, *Anatomia Histologia Embryologia,* 2000, 29:321–329.

CASALE SA, MCCARTHY RJ, Complications associated with lateral fabellotibial suture surgery for cranial cruciate ligament injury in dogs: 363 cases (1997–2005), *Journal of the American Veterinary Medical Association,* 2009, 234:229–235.

CASHMORE RG et al., Major complications and risk factors associated with surgical correction of congenital medial patellar luxation in 124 dogs, *Veterinary and Comparative Orthopaedics and Traumatology,* 2014, 27:263–270.

CHAILLEUX N et al., In vitro 3-dimensional kinematic evaluation of 2 corrective operations for cranial cruciate ligament-deficient stifle, *Canadian Journal of Veterinary Research,* 2007, 71:175–180.

CHAUVET AE et al., Evaluation of fibular head transposition, lateral fabellar suture, and conservative treatment of cranial cruciate ligament rupture in large dogs: a retrospective study, *Journal of the American Animal Hospital Association,* 1996, 32:247–255.

CINTI F et al., Two different approaches for novel extracapsular cranial cruciate ligament reconstruction: an in vitro kinematics study, *Journal of Small Animal Practice,* 2015, 56:398–406.

COLETTI TJ et al., Complications associated with tibial plateau leveling osteotomy: a retrospective of 1519 procedures, *Canadian Veterinary Journal,* 2014, 55:249–254.

COLLINS JE et al., Benefits of pre- and intraoperative planning for tibial plateau leveling osteotomy, *Veterinary Surgery,* 2014, 43(2):142–149.

COMERFORD E et al., Management of cranial cruciate ligament injury in small dogs: a questionnaire study, *Veterinary and Comparative Orthopaedics and Traumatology,* 2013, 26:493–497.

Conkling AL, Fagin B, Daye RM, Comparison of tibial plateau angle changes after tibial plateau leveling osteotomy fixation with conventional or locking screw technology, *Veterinary Surgery*, 2010, 39(4):475–481.

Conzemius MG et al., Effect of surgical technique on limb function after surgery for rupture of the cranial cruciate ligament in dogs, *Journal of the American Veterinary Medical Association*, 2005, 226:232–236.

Cook JL et al., Clinical comparison of a novel extracapsular stabilization procedure and tibial plateau leveling osteotomy for treatment of cranial cruciate ligament deficiency in dogs, *Veterinary Surgery*, 2010, 39(3):315–323.

Corr SA, Brown C, A comparison of outcomes following tibial plateau levelling osteotomy and cranial tibial wedge osteotomy procedures, *Veterinary and Comparative Orthopaedics and Traumatology*, 2007, 20:312–319.

Cosenza G, Reif U, Martini FM, Tibial plateau levelling osteotomy in 69 small breed dogs using conically coupled 1.9/2.5 mm locking plates. A clinical and radiographic retrospective assessment. *Veterinary and Comparative Orthopaedics and Traumatology*, 2015, 28:347–354.

Cox JS, Cordell LD, The degenerative effects of medial meniscus tears in dogs' knees, *Clinical Orthopaedics and Related Research*, 1977, 125:236–242.

De Sousa R et al., Treatment of cranial cruciate ligament rupture in the feline stifle, *Veterinary and Comparative Orthopaedics and Traumatology*, 2015, 28:401–408.

De Sousa RJ et al., Quasi-isometric points for the technique of lateral suture placement in the feline stifle joint, *Veterinary Surgery*, 2014, 43(2):120–126.

Dillon DE et al., Risk factors and diagnostic accuracy of clinical findings for meniscal disease in dogs with cranial cruciate ligament disease, *Veterinary Surgery*, 2014, 43(4):446–450.

Duerr FM et al., Comparison of surgical treatment options for cranial cruciate ligament disease in large-breed dogs with excessive tibial plateau angle, *Veterinary Surgery*, 2008, 37(1):49–62.

Duerr FM et al., Treatment of canine cranial cruciate ligament disease, *Veterinary and Comparative Orthopaedics and Traumatology*, 2014, 27:478–483.

Duval JM et al., Breed, sex, and bodyweight as risk factors for rupture of the cranial cruciate ligament in young dogs, *Journal of the American Veterinary Medical Association*, 1999, 6:811–814.

Dymond NL, Goldsmid SE, Simpson DJ, Tibial tuberosity advancement in 92 canine stifles: initial results, clinical outcome and owner evaluation, *Australian Veterinary Journal*, 2010, 88(10):381–385.

Ertelt J, Fehr M, Cranial cruciate ligament repair in dogs with and without meniscal lesions treated by different minimally invasive methods, *Veterinary and Comparative Orthopaedics and Traumatology*, 2009, 22(1):21–26.

Farrell M et al., Ex vivo evaluation of the effect of tibial plateau osteotomy on the proximal tibial soft tissue envelope with and without the use of protective gauze sponges, *Veterinary Surgery*, 2009, 38(5):636–644.

Farrell M et al., In vitro performance testing of two arcuate oscillating saw blades designed for use during tibial plateau leveling osteotomy, *Veterinary Surgery*, 2011, 40(6):694–707.

Fitzpatrick N, Solano MA, Predictive variables for complications after TPLO with stifle inspection by arthrotomy in 1000 consecutive dogs, *Veterinary Surgery*, 2010, 39(4):460–474.

Flo GL, Meniscal injuries, *Veterinary Clinics of North America: Small Animal Practice*, 1993, 23:831–843.

Flo GL, Modification of the lateral retinacular imbrication technique for stabilizing cruciate ligament injuries, *Journal of the American Animal Hospital Association*, 1975, 11:570–576.

Fossum TW, *Small Animal Surgery*, 3rd edition, 2007, Mosby.

Franklin SP, Gilley RS, Palmer RH, Meniscal injury in dogs with cranial cruciate ligament rupture, *Compendium on Continuing Education for the Practising Veterinarian*, 2010, 32(10):E1-10, quiz E11.

Gallagher AD, Mertens WD, Implant removal rate from infection after tibial plateau leveling osteotomy in dogs, *Veterinary Surgery*, 2012, 41(6):705–711.

Gallegos J et al., Postoperative complications and short-term outcome following single-session bilateral corrective surgery for medial patellar luxation in dogs weighing <15 kg: 50 cases (2009–2014), *Veterinary Surgery*, 2016, 45(7):887–892.

Gatineau M et al., Retrospective study of tibial plateau levelling osteotomy procedures. Rate of subsequent 'pivot shift', meniscal tear and other complications, *Veterinary and Comparative Orthopaedics and Traumatology*, 2011, 24:333–341.

Gonzalo-Orden JM et al., Magnetic resonance imaging in 50 dogs with stifle lameness, *European Journal of Companion Animal Practice*, 2001, 11:115–118.

GORDON-EVANS WJ et al., Comparison of lateral fabellar suture and tibial plateau leveling osteotomy techniques for treatment of dogs with cranial cruciate ligament disease, *Journal of the American Veterinary Medical Association*, 2013, 24(3):675–680.

GRIFFON DJ, A review of the pathogenesis of canine cranial cruciate ligament disease as a basis for future preventive strategies, *Veterinary Surgery*, 2010, 39(4):399–409.

HANS EC et al., Outcome following surgical correction of grade 4 medial patellar luxation in dogs: 47 stifles (2001–2012), *Journal of the American Animal Hospital Association*, 2016, 52:162–169.

HARPER TA et al., Sensitivity of low-field T2 images for detecting the presence and severity of histopathologic meniscal lesions in dogs, *Veterinary Radiology and Ultrasound*, 2011, 52:428–435.

HART JL et al., Comparison of owner satisfaction between stifle joint orthoses and tibial plateau leveling osteotomy for the management of cranial cruciate ligament disease in dogs, *Journal of the American Veterinary Medical Association*, 2016, 249:391–398.

HAYES GM et al., Abnormal reflex activation of hamstring muscles in dogs with cranial cruciate ligament rupture, *The Veterinary Journal*, 2013, 196:345–350.

HAYES GM, LANGLEY-HOBBS SJ, JEFFERY ND, Risk factors for medial meniscal injury in association with cranial cruciate ligament rupture, *Journal of Small Animal Practice*, 2010, 51:630–634.

HULSE D et al., Determination of isometric points for placement of a lateral suture in treatment of the cranial cruciate ligament deficient stifle, *Veterinary and Comparative Orthopaedics and Traumatology*, 2010a, 23:163–167.

HULSE D, BEALE B, KERWIN S, Second look arthroscopic findings after tibial plateau leveling osteotomy, *Veterinary Surgery*, 2010b, 39(3):350–354.

HULSE D, JOHNSON S. Isolated lateral meniscal tear in the dog, *Veterinary and Comparative Orthopaedics and Traumatology*, 1998, 3:152–154.

INNES JF et al., Long-term outcome of surgery for dogs with cranial cruciate ligament deficiency, *Veterinary Record*, 2000, 147:325–328.

JERRAM RM, WALKER AM, WARMAN CG, Proximal tibial intraarticular ostectomy for treatment of canine cranial cruciate ligament injury, *Veterinary Surgery*, 2005, 34(3):196–205.

JOHNSON AL et al., Comparison of trochlear block recession and trochlear wedge recession for canine patellar luxation using a cadaver model, *Veterinary Surgery*, 2001, 30(2):140–150.

JOHNSON JA, AUSTIN C, BREUR GJ, Incidence of canine appendicular musculoskeletal disorders in 16 veterinary teaching hospitals from 1980 through 1989, *Veterinary and Comparative Orthopaedics and Traumatology*, 1994, 7:56–69.

JOHNSON KA, *Piermattei's Atlas of Surgical Approaches to the Bones and Joints of the Dog and Cat,* 5th ed., Saint Louis, Elsevier-Saunders, 2014, p. 488.

JOHNSON KA et al., Comparison of the effects of caudal pole hemi-meniscectomy and complete medial meniscectomy in the canine stifle joint, *American Journal of Veterinary Research,* 2004, 65:1053–1060.

KALFF S, MEACHEM S, PRESTON C, Incidence of medial meniscal tears after arthroscopic assisted tibial plateau leveling osteotomy, *Veterinary Surgery*, 2011, 40(8):952–956.

KALFF S et al., Lateral patellar luxation in dogs: a retrospective study of 65 dogs, *Veterinary and Comparative Orthopaedics and Traumatology*, 2014, 27:130–134.

KENNEDY SC et al., The effect of axial and abaxial release on meniscal displacement in the dog, *Veterinary and Comparative Orthopaedics and Traumatology*, 2005, 18:227–234.

KIM SE et al., Effect of tibial plateau leveling osteotomy on femorotibial contact mechanics and stifle kinematics, *Veterinary Surgery*, 2009, 38(1):23–32.

KRAYER M et al., Apoptosis of ligamentous cells of the cranial cruciate ligament from stable stifle joints of dogs with partial cranial cruciate ligament rupture, *American Journal of Veterinary Research*, 2008, 69:625–630.

KROTSCHECK U et al., Long term functional outcome of tibial tuberosity advancement vs. tibial plateau leveling osteotomy and extracapsular repair in a heterogeneous population of dogs, *Veterinary Surgery*, 2016, 45(2):261–268.

KUAN S, SMITH B, BLACK A, Tibial wedge ostectomy: complications of 300 surgical procedures, *Australian Veterinary Journal*, 2009, 87(11):438–444.

LAFAVER S et al., Tibial tuberosity advancement for stabilization of the cranial cruciate ligament-deficient stifle joint: surgical technique, early results, and complications in 101 dogs, *Veterinary Surgery*, 2007, 36(6):573–586.

LANGLEY-HOBBS SJ, Lateral meniscal tears and stifle osteochondrosis in three dogs, *Veterinary Record*, 2001, 149:592–594.

Leighton RL, Preferred method of repair of cranial cruciate ligament rupture in dogs: a survey of ACVS diplomates specializing in canine orthopedics, American College of Veterinary Surgery. *Veterinary Surgery*, 1999, 28(3):194.

Mahn MM et al., Arthroscopic verification of ultrasonographic diagnosis of meniscal pathology in dogs, *Veterinary Surgery*, 2005, 34(4):318–323.

McCready DJM, Ness MG, Diagnosis and management of meniscal injury in dogs with cranial and cruciate ligament rupture: a systematic literature review, *Journal of Small Animal Practice*, 2016, 57:59–66.

Mindner JK et al., Tibial plateau levelling osteotomy in eleven cats with cranial cruciate ligament rupture, *Veterinary and Comparative Orthopaedics and Traumatology*, 2016, 29:528–535.

Monk ML, Preston CA, Mcgowan CM, Effects of early intensive postoperative physiotherapy on limb function after tibial plateau leveling osteotomy in dogs with deficiency of the cranial cruciate ligament, *American Journal of Veterinary Research*, 2006, 67:529–536.

Montavon PM, Tibial tuberosity advancement TTA for cranial cruciate ligament disease, *Proceedings of the World Small Animal Veterinary Association World Congress*, 2010, Geneva, Switzerland.

Montavon PM, Damur DM, Tepic S, Advancement of the tibial tuberosity for the treatment of cranial cruciate deficient canine stifle, *Proceedings of the 1st World Veterinary Orthopaedic Congress*, 2002 September 5–8, Munich, Germany, p. 89.

Mostafa AA et al., Proximodistal alignment of the canine patella: radiographic evaluation and association with medial and lateral patellar luxation, *Veterinary Surgery*, 2008, 37(3):201–211.

Morgan JP et al., Correlation of radiographic changes after tibial tuberosity advancement in dogs with cranial cruciate-deficient stifles with functional outcome, *Veterinary Surgery*, 2010, 39(4):425–432.

Muro NM, Lanz OI, Use of a novel extracapsular bone anchor system for stabilisation of cranial cruciate ligament insufficiency, *Journal of Small Animal Practice*, 2017, 58(5):284–292.

Murphy S et al., A randomized prospective comparison of dogs undergoing tibial tuberosity advancement or tibial plateau leveling osteotomy for cranial cruciate ligament rupture, *Proceedings of the 17th ESVOT Congress*, 2014, 2–4 October, Venice, Italy.

Neal BA et al., Evaluation of meniscal click for detecting meniscal tears in stifles with cranial cruciate ligament disease, *Veterinary Surgery*, 2015, 44(2):191–194.

Nelson SA et al., Long-term functional outcome of tibial plateau leveling osteotomy versus extracapsular repair in a heterogeneous population of dogs, *Veterinary Surgery*, 2013, 42(1):38–50.

Ness MG et al., A survey of orthopaedic conditions in small animal veterinary practice in Britain, *Veterinary and Comparative Orthopaedics and Traumatology*, 1996, 9:43–52.

O'Brien CS, Martinez SA, Potential iatrogenic medial meniscal damage during tibial plateau leveling osteotomy, *Veterinary Surgery*, 2009, 38(7):868–873.

Olive J et al., Fast presurgical magnetic resonance imaging of meniscal tears and concurrent subchondral bone marrow lesions: study of dogs with naturally occurring cranial cruciate ligament rupture, *Veterinary and Comparative Orthopaedics and Traumatology*, 2014, 27:1–7.

Olmstead ML, The use of orthopedic wire as a lateral suture for stifle stabilization, *Veterinary Clinics of North America: Small Animal Practice*, 1993, 23:735–753.

Oxley B et al., Precision of a novel computed tomographic method for quantification of femoral varus in dogs and an assessment of the effect of femoral malpositioning, *Veterinary Surgery*, 2013a, 42:751–758.

Oxley B.et al., Comparison of complication rates and clinical outcome between tibial plateau leveling osteotomy and a modified cranial closing wedge osteotomy for treatment of cranial cruciate ligament disease in dogs, *Veterinary Surgery*, 2013b, 42(6):739–750.

Pacchiana PD et al., Surgical and postoperative complications associated with tibial plateau leveling osteotomy in dogs with cranial cruciate ligament rupture: 397 cases (1998–2001), *Journal of the American Veterinary Medical Association*, 2003, 222:184–193.

Petazzoni M, Jaeger GH, *Atlas of Clinical Goniometry and Radiographic Measurements of the Canine Pelvic Limb* 2nd ed., 2008 Merial, Duluth.

Plesman R, Gilbert P, Campbell J, Detection of meniscal tears by arthroscopy and arthrotomy in dogs with cranial cruciate ligament rupture. A retrospective cohort study, *Veterinary and Comparative Orthopaedics and Traumatology*, 2013, 1:42–46.

Pozzi A, Hildreth BE 3rd, Rajala-Schultz PJ, Comparison of arthroscopy and arthrotomy for diagnosis of medial meniscal pathology: an ex vivo study, *Veterinary Surgery*, 2008, 37(8):749–755.

Pozzi A, Kim SE, Lewis DD, Effect of transection of the caudal menisco-tibial ligament on medial femorotibial contact mechanics, *Veterinary Surgery*, 2010, 39(4):489–495.

Pozzi A, Samii V, Horodyski MB, Evaluation of vascular trauma after tibial plateau levelling osteotomy with or without gauze protection. A cadaveric angiographic study, *Veterinary and Comparative Orthopaedics and Traumatology*, 2011, 24:266–271.

Priddy NH 2nd et al., Complications with and owner assessment of the outcome of tibial plateau leveling osteotomy for treatment of cranial cruciate ligament rupture in dogs: 193 cases (1997–2001), *Journal of the American Veterinary Medical Association*, 2003, 222:1726–1732.

Putnam RW, *Patellar Luxation in the Dog,* 1968, Master of Science Thesis, University of Guelph, Ontario.

Ralphs SC, Whitney WO, Arthroscopic evaluation of menisci in dogs with cranial cruciate ligament injuries: 100 cases (1999–2000), *Journal of the American Veterinary Medical Association,* 2002, 221:1601–1604.

Rayward RM et al., Progression of osteoarthritis following TPLO surgery: a prospective radiographic study of 40 dogs, *Journal of Small Animal Practice*, 2004, 45(2):92–97.

Remedios AM et al., Medial patellar luxation in 16 large dogs. A retrospective study, *Veterinary Surgery*, 1992, 21(1):5–9.

Robinson DA et al., The effect of tibial plateau angle on ground reaction forces 4–17 months after tibial plateau leveling osteotomy in Labrador Retrievers, *Veterinary Surgery*, 2006, 35(3):294–299.

Roush JK, Canine patellar luxation, *Veterinary Clinics of North America: Small Animal Practice*, 1993, 23:855–868.

Rutherford S, Bell JC, Ness MG, Fracture of the patella after TPLO in 6 dogs, *Veterinary Surgery*, 2012, 41(7):869–875.

Schmerbach KI et al., In vitro comparison of tibial plateau leveling osteotomy with and without use of a tibial plateau leveling jig, *Veterinary Surgery*, 2007, 36(2):156–163.

Segal U, Or M, Shani J, Latero-distal transposition of the tibial crest in cases of medial patellar luxation with patella alta, *Veterinary and Comparative Orthopaedics and Traumatology*, 2012, 25(4):281–285.

Slocum B, Devine T, The knee. In: *Current Techniques in Small Animal Surgery,* Bojrab MJ, Ellison GW, Slocum B (eds.), Philadelphia, Williams and Wilkins, 1998, pp. 1187–1244.

Slocum B, Slocum TD, Tibial plateau leveling osteotomy for repair of cranial cruciate ligament rupture in the canine, *Veterinary Clinics of North America: Small Animal Practice*, 1993, 23:777–795.

Slocum B, Devine T, Cranial tibial wedge osteotomy: a technique for eliminating cranial tibial thrust in cranial cruciate ligament repair, *Journal of the American Veterinary Medical Association*, 1984, 184(5):564–569.

Smith T et al., Tibial plateau levelling osteotomy in an alpaca, *Veterinary and Comparative Orthopaedics and Traumatology*, 2009, 22:332–335.

Smith GK, Torg JS, Fibular head transposition for repair of cruciate-deficient stifle in the dog, *Journal of the American Veterinary Medical Association*, 1985, 187(4):375–383.

Solano MA et al., Locking plate and screw fixation after tibial plateau leveling osteotomy reduces postoperative infection rate in dogs over 50 kg, *Veterinary Surgery*, 2015, 44(1):59–64.

Soparat C et al., Radiographic measurement for femoral varus in Pomeranian dogs with and without medial patellar luxation, *Veterinary and Comparative Orthopaedics and Traumatology*, 2012, 253:197–201.

Stein S, Schmoekel HJ, Short-term and eight to 12 months results of a tibial tuberosity advancement as treatment of canine cranial cruciate ligament damage, *Journal of Small Animal Practice*, 2008 49(8):398–404.

Taylor-Brown F et al., Magnetic resonance imaging for detection of late meniscal tears in dogs following tibial tuberosity advancement for treatment of cranial cruciate ligament injury, *Veterinary and Comparative Orthopaedics and Traumatology*, 2014, 27:141–146.

Tepic S, Montavon PM, Is cranial tibial advancement relevant in the cruciate deficient stifle? *Proceedings of the 12th ESVOT Congress*, 2004 September 10–12, Munich, Germany, pp. 132–133.

Thieman KM et al., Effect of meniscal release on rate of subsequent meniscal tears and owner-assessed outcome in dogs with cruciate disease treated with tibial plateau leveling osteotomy, *Veterinary Surgery*, 2006, 35(8):705–710.

Tivers MS et al., Diagnostic accuracy of positive contrast computed tomography arthrography for the detection of injuries to the medial meniscus in dogs with naturally occurring cranial cruciate ligament insufficiency, *Journal of Small Animal Practice*, 2009, 50:324–332.

Tobias KM, Johnston SA, *Veterinary Surgery: Small Animal*, 2nd edition, 2017, Saint Louis, Elsevier-Saunders.

Tonks CA et al., The effects of extra-articular suture tension on contact mechanics of the lateral compartment of cadaveric stifles treated with the TightRope CCL or lateral suture technique, *Veterinary Surgery*, 2010, 39(3):343–349.

TONKS CA, LEWIS DD, POZZI A, A review of extra-articular prosthetic stabilization of the cranial cruciate ligament-deficient stifle, *Veterinary and Comparative Orthopaedics and Traumatology*, 2011, 24:167–177.

TUTTLE TA, MANLEY PA, Risk factors associated with fibular fracture after tibial plateau leveling osteotomy, *Veterinary Surgery*, 2009, 38(3):355–360.

VALEN S et al., A modified compression test for the detectipon of meniscal injury in dogs, *Journal of Small Animal Practice*, 2017, 58:109–114.

VASSEUR PB, The stifle joint. In: *Textbook of Small Animal Surgery, Volume 2*, 2nd ed., SLATTER DH (ed.), Philadelphia, Saunders, 1993, pp. 1817–1866.

VASSEUR PB, Clinical results following nonoperative management for rupture of the cranial cruciate ligament in dogs, *Veterinary Surgery*, 1984, 13(4):243–246.

VOSS K et al., Force plate gait analysis to assess limb function after tibial tuberosity advancement in dogs with cranial cruciate ligament disease, *Veterinary and Comparative Orthopaedics and Traumatology*, 2008, 21(3):243–249.

WALLACE AM et al., Modification of the cranial closing wedge ostectomy technique for the treatment of canine cruciate disease. Description and comparison with standard technique, *Veterinary and Comparative Orthopaedics and Traumatology*, 2011, 24(6):457–62.

WARZEE CC et al., Effect of tibial plateau leveling on cranial and caudal tibial thrusts in canine cranial cruciate–deficient stifles: an in vitro experimental study, *Veterinary Surgery*, 2001, 30(3):278–286.

WHITNEY WO, Arthroscopically assisted surgery of the stifle joint. In: *Small Animal Arthroscopy*, BEALE BS, HULSE DA, SCHULZ KS, WHITNEY WO, Philadelphia, Saunders, 2003, pp. 137–140.

WILKE VL et al., Estimate of the annual economic impact of treatment of cranial cruciate ligament injury in dogs in the United States, *Journal of the American Veterinary Medical Association*, 2005, 227:1604–1607.

WILLIAMS RA, Isolated meniscal tear in a Boxer, *Veterinary Record*, 2010, 167:419–420.

WITSBERGER TH et al., Prevalence of and risk factors for hip dysplasia and cranial cruciate ligament deficiency in dogs, *Journal of the American Veterinary Medical Association*, 2008, 232:1818–1824.

WITTE PG, Tibial anatomy in normal small breed dogs including anisometry of various extracapsular stabilizing suture attachment sites, *Veterinary and Comparative Orthopaedics and Traumatology*, 2015, 28:331–338.

WITTE PG, SCOTT HW, Tibial plateau leveling osteotomy in small breed dogs with high tibial plateau angles using a 4-hole 1.9/2.5 mm locking T-plate, *Veterinary Surgery*, 2014, 43(5):549–557.

WUCHERER KL et al., Short-term and long-term outcomes for overweight dogs with cranial cruciate ligament rupture treated surgically or nonsurgically, *Journal of the American Veterinary Medical Association*, 2013, 242:1364–1372.

CHAPTER 3

ALLAN RM, A modified Maquet technique for management of cranial cruciate avulsion in a cat, *Journal of Small Animal Practice,* 2014, 55(1):52–56.

ARON DN, PURINTON TP, Collateral ligaments of the tarsocrural joint: an anatomical and functional study, *Veterinary Surgery,* 1985a, 14(3):173–177.

ARON DN, PURINTON TP, Replacement of the collateral ligaments of the canine tarsocrural joint: a proposed technique, *Veterinary Surgery,* 1985b, 14(3):178–184.

BALTZER WI, RIST P, Achilles tendon repair in dogs using the semitendinosus muscle: surgical technique and short-term outcome in five dogs, *Veterinary Surgery*, 2009, 38(6):770–779.

BARNES DC et al., Complications of lateral plate fixation compared with tension band wiring and pin or lag screw fixation for calcaneoquartal arthrodesis, *Veterinary and Comparative Orthopaedics and Traumatology*, 2013, 26(6):445–452.

BEARDSLEY SL, SCHRADER SC, Treatment of dogs with wounds of the limbs caused by shearing forces: 98 cases (1975–1993), *Journal of the American Veterinary Medical Association*, 1995, 207(8):1071–1075.

BEEVER LJ, KULENDRA ET, MEESON RL, Short and long-term outcome following surgical stabilization of tarsocrural instability in dogs. *Veterinary and Comparative Orthopaedics and Traumatology*, 2016, 29(2):142–148.

BOJRAB MJ, WALDRON DR, TOOMBS JP, *Current Techniques in Small Animal Surgery*, 5th ed., Jackson, Wyoming, Teton NewMedia, 2014, pp. 1092–1118

CASE JB et al., Gastrocnemius tendon strain in a dog treated with autologous mesenchymal stem cells and a custom orthosis, *Veterinary Surgery,* 2013, 42(4):355–360.

CERVI M, BREBNER, N, LIPTAK, J, Short- and long-term outcomes of primary Achilles tendon repair in cats: 21 Cases. *Veterinary and Comparative Orthopaedics and Traumatology*, 2010, 23(5):348–353.

CORR S, Intensive, extensive, expensive: management of distal limb shearing injuries in cats, *Journal of Feline Medicine and Surgery*, 2009, 11(9):747–757.

CORR SA et al., Retrospective study of Achilles mechanism disruption in 45 dogs. *The Veterinary Record*, 2010, 167(11):407–411.

DECAMP, CE et al., *Brinker, Piermattei and Flo's Handbook Of Small Animal Orthopedics And Fracture Repair*, 5th ed., Saint Louis, Elsevier-Saunders, 2016, pp. 707–758.

DIAMOND DW, BESSO J, BOUDRIEAU, RJ, Evaluation of joint stabilization for treatment of shearing injuries of the tarsus in 20 dogs. *Journal of the American Animal Hospital Association*, 1999, 35(2):147–153.

DISERENS KA, VENZIN C, Chronic Achilles tendon rupture augmented by transposition of the fibularis brevis and fibularis longus muscles, *Schweizer Archiv für Tierheilkunde*, 2015, 157(9):519–524.

HOFFER MJ et al., Clinical applications of demineralized bone matrix: a retrospective and case-matched study of seventy-five dogs, *Veterinary Surgery*, 2008, 37(7):639–647.

JAEGER GH et al., Use of hinged transarticular external fixation for adjunctive joint stabilization in dogs and cats: 14 cases (1999–2003), *Journal of the American Veterinary Medical Association*, 2005, 227(4):586–591.

JAEGER GH et al., Validity of goniometric joint measurements in cats. *American Journal of Veterinary Research*, 2007, 68(8):822–826.

JAEGGER G, MARCELLIN-LITTLE DJ, Reliability of goniometry in Labrador Retrievers. *American Journal of Veterinary Research*, 2002, 63(7):979–986.

JOHNSON A, HOULTON J, VANNINI R, *AO Principles of Fracture Management in the Dog and Cat*, New York, Thieme, 2005.

JOHNSON KA, *Piermattei's Atlas of Surgical Approaches to the Bones and Joints of the Dog and Cat*, 5th ed., St Louis, Elsevier-Saunders, 2014, pp. 440–459

KRAUS KH, TOOMBS JP, NESS MG, *External Fixation in Small Animal Practice*, Oxford, Blackwell Publishing, 2008, pp. 1–232.

KULENDRA E et al., Evaluation of the transarticular external skeletal fixator for the treatment of tarsocrural instability in 32 cats, *Veterinary and Comparative Orthopaedics and Traumatology*, 2011, 24(5):320–325.

MCKEE WM et al., Pantarsal arthrodesis with a customised medial or lateral bone plate in 13 dogs, *The Veterinary Record*, 2004, 154(6):165–170.

MEESON RL, DAVIDSON C, ARTHURS GI, Soft-tissue injuries associated with cast application for distal limb orthopaedic conditions, A retrospective study of sixty dogs and cats, *Veterinary and Comparative Orthopaedics and Traumatology*, 2011, 24(2):126–131.

MEUTSTEGE FJ, The classification of canine Achilles' tendon lesions, *Veterinary and Comparative Orthopaedics and Traumatology*, 1993: 6(1):57–59.

MONTAVON PM, VOSS K, LANGLEY-HOBBS SJ, *Feline Orthopedic Surgery and Musculoskeletal Disease*, Edinburgh, Saunders Limited, 2009, pp. 507–525.

MILLER ME, EVANS HE, DE LAHUNTA A, *Miller's Anatomy of the Dog*, St Louis, Elsevier, 2013, various chapters.

MOORES AP et al., Biomechanical and clinical evaluation of a modified 3-loop pulley suture pattern for reattachment of canine tendons to bone, *Veterinary Surgery*, 2004a, 33(4):391–397.

MOORES AP, OWEN MR, TARLTON JF, The three-loop pulley suture versus two locking-loop sutures for the repair of canine Achilles tendons, *Veterinary Surgery*, 2004b, 33(2):131–137.

Morton MA et al., Repair of chronic rupture of the insertion of the gastrocnemius tendon in the dog using a polyethylene terephthalate implants, *Veterinary and Comparative Orthopaedics and Traumatology*, 2015, 28(4):282–287.

Nielsen C, Pluhar GE, Outcome following surgical repair of Achilles tendon rupture and comparison between postoperative tibiotarsal immobilization methods in dogs – 28 cases (1997–2004), *Veterinary and Comparative Orthopaedics and Traumatology,* 2006, 19(4):246–249.

Roch SP et al., Complications following tarsal arthrodesis using bone plate fixation in dogs. *Journal of Small Animal Practice*, 2008, 49(3):117–126.

Schmökel HG et al., Tarsal injuries in the cat: A retrospective study of 21 cases, *Journal of Small Animal Practice,* 1994, 35(3):156–162.

Sivacolundhu RK et al., Achilles mechanism reconstruction in four dogs, *Veterinary and Comparative Orthopaedics and Traumatology*, 2001, 14(1):25–31.

Swaim SF, Welch JA, Gillette RL, *Management of Small Animal Distal Limb Injuries*, Jackson, Wyoming, Tenon NewMedia, 2015, pp. 1–392.

Swiderski J et al., Sonographic assisted diagnosis and treatment of bilateral gastrocnemius tendon rupture in a Labrador retriever repaired with fascia lata and polypropylene mesh. *Veterinary and Comparative Orthopaedics and Traumatology*, 2005, 18(4):258–263.

Tobias KM, Johnston SA, *Veterinary Surgery: Small Animal: Volume I*, St Louis, Elsevier, 2013, pp. 1014–1028.

Tomlinson J, Moore R, Locking loop tendon suture use in repair of five calcanean tendons, *Veterinary Surgery*, 1982, 11:105–109.